THE IMAGING OF INFECTION AND INFLAMMATION

Developments in Nuclear Medicine

VOLUME 31

Series Editor: Peter H. Cox

The Imaging of Infection and Inflammation

edited by

PETER H. COX

Department of Nuclear Medicine,
Dr Daniel den Hoed Cancer Center,
University Hospital Rotterdam, The Netherlands

and

JOHN R. BUSCOMBE

Department of Nuclear Medicine,
Royal Free Hospital, London, U.K.

KLUWER ACADEMIC PUBLISHERS
DORDRECHT / BOSTON / LONDON

A C.I.P. Catalogue record for this book is available from the Library of Congress.

ISBN 0-7923-5087-1

Published by Kluwer Academic Publishers,
P.O. Box 17, 3300 AA Dordrecht, The Netherlands.

Sold and distributed in the North, Central and South America
by Kluwer Academic Publishers,
101 Philip Drive, Norwell, MA 02061, U.S.A.

In all other countries, sold and distributed
by Kluwer Academic Publishers,
P.O. Box 322, 3300 AH Dordrecht, The Netherlands.

Printed on acid-free paper

Printed in the Netherlands.

TABLE OF CONTENTS

List of Contributors

R. Baker
Academic Infectious Disease Unit, University College London Medical School. Windeyer Building Room G41, 46 Cleveland Street, London W1P 6DB, UK

W. Becker
Abteilung für Nuklearmedizin, Zentrum Radiologie, Universität Göttingen, Robert-Koch Strasse 40, D-37075 Göttingen, Germany

P.J. Blower
Department of Nuclear Medicine, Kent and Canterbury Hospital, Canterbury CT1 3NG, UK

J.R. Buscombe
Department of Nuclear Medicine, Royal Free Hospital, Pond Street, London NW3 2QG, UK

D.P. Clarke
Department of Nuclear Medicine, Royal Free Hospital, Pond Street, London NW3 2QG, UK

P.H. Cox
Department of Nuclear Medicine, Dr Daniel den Hoed Cancer Centre, University Hospital Rotterdam, P.O. Box, 5210 3008 AE Rotterdam, The Netherlands

M.J. O'Doherty
Department of Nuclear Medicine, St Thomas' Hospital, London SE1 7EH, UK

R. Kashyap
Department of Nuclear Medicine, St Bartholomew's Hospital, West Smithfield, London EC1A 7BE, UK

A.M. Peters
Department of Diagnostic Radiology, Royal Postgraduate Medical School, Hammersmith Hospital, DuCane Road, London W12 0NN, UK

C.B. Sampson
Department of Nuclear Medicine, Addenbrookes Hospital, Cambridge CB2 2QQ, UK

M.J. Weldon
Department of Biochemical Medicine, St Georges Hospital Medical School, Cranmer Terrace, London SW7 0RE, UK

FOREWORD

Despite the advances which have been made in the development of therapeutic drugs infection remains one of the major health problems world wide. The development of drug resistant strains of bacteria and parasites serves to enhance this problem. Diagnostic medical procedures play a major role in the identification of foci of infection and in differentiating between infection and sterile inflammation. The development of radiopharmaceuticals based upon biologically active carrier molecules such as antibodies and peptides offers new opportunities to introduce more specific diagnostic agents to complement CT, MRI and Ultrasound.

This volume reviews the state of the art with respect to nuclear medical procedures for the detection of infection and inflammation and discusses future developments in this field.
The Editors would like to acknowledge the assistance of Mrs T. Busker and T. Klijn in preparing the written text and Mrs M. Cox-King for her help in preparing the layout.

"At the time of going to press news reached us of the untimely death of one of our contributors Mr Charles Sampson. Charles was well known and respected for this contributions to Radiopharmacy which earned him an international reputation but in addition was a gifted violinist who also made a significant contributon to the world of music. He will be greatly missed. P.H.C."

P.H.C.
Rotterdam 1998.

CHAPTER 1

INFECTION IN HOSPITALS

R. Baker, A. Zumla, B.S. Peters

Introduction

Infectious Disease is a clinical speciality which crosses the boundaries of all other medical disciplines. Hippocrates and Galen were able to diagnose typhoid and malaria by the characteristic pattern of their fevers. Most infectious and inflammatory conditions however do not have such diagnostic clinical features. The accurate localisation and characterisation of inflammation and infection has emerged as one of the greatest challenges of modern medicine. This challenge is increased by the advent of large numbers of patients with profound immunosuppression, either due to AIDS or iatrogenically during chemotherapy. Immunosuppressed patients may have severe infection without exhibiting any of the classical signs and symptoms. Furthermore the introduction of an ever increasing range of invasive procedures has led to a greater incidence and diversity of infective sequelae.

Finally, as the current millenium draws to a close we are in danger of returning to the pre-antibiotic era for some infections. There is only one drug at present consistently effective against MRSA, a strain of enterococcus has emerged which is resistant to vancomycin and a form of Tuberculosis resistant to multiple drugs has emerged.

Infection amongst the Elderly

The aging of the population has focused attention on the special needs of elderly patients [1]. The aged do not tend to mount the same degree of fevers or leucocytosis, or have the intensity of symptoms and signs in response to infection as younger people [2]. Age associated impairment of immunity, such as reduced T-cell activity and IL-2 production, are associated with an increased morbidity from and increased reactivation of latent infection [3]. Cell mediated and humoral immunity is attenuated [4], wounds do not heal so rapidly [5], and there may be other problems associated with diminished mobility and poorer circulation. The generally unwell, confused elderly patient with infection is a very frequent problem in both hospital and the community [6].

1

P. H.Cox and J. R. Buscombe (eds.), The Imaging of Infection and Inflammation, 1–19.
© 1998 Kluwer Academic Publishers. Printed in the Netherlands.

Both asymptomatic bacteruria and true urinary tract infection are increased [7] and upper urinary tract infections are more likely to be fatal. Urinary catheters readily introduce infection. Diarrhoeal illness is more common particularly in institutions, and may lead to death, [8]. Concomitant antibiotic treatment, gut pathology or achlorhydria may contribute to an increased susceptibility to infection particularly with *Salmonella* spp. Pneumonia is more common in the elderly than for any other age range - 97% of all community acquired or nosocomial deaths due to pneumonia occur in this group [9]. The proportions of the infecting organisms are different: influenza is less common, whereas respiratory syncitial virus, gram negative bacilli and *S. Aureus* are more common than in younger individuals [10]. Diminished cough reflex may make sputum collection more difficult and aspiration more likely. Age alone however does not predict mortality [11]. More important is the presence of other illness. Tuberculosis is more common in the elderly [12]. The largest reservoir of tuberculous infection in Europe is the white indigenous over-55 population who are becoming immunodecrepit, and whose endogenous infection reactivates.

Infected pressure sores are a major problem in the debilitated and immobile elderly person. A particular problem is differentiating skin commensals from pathogenic organisms. Lesions may be slow to heal, there may be underlying osteomyelitis and bacteraemia may result. Bacteraemia generally is more common in both extremes of age and more likely to lead to death [13,14]. Infections of the urogenital, gastrointestinal and respiratory tracts are the most likely sources [15,16]. The decreased incidence of rheumatic heart disease in the young has meant that bacterial endocarditis is more and more a disease of the elderly, who have more non-specific symptoms than do younger patients [17]. Meningitis in the elderly may have a less florid presentation and is likely to be fatal. In recent years there has been a much larger proportion of aged individuals with prosthetic joints which subsequently can become infected[18].

Patients with Malignant Disease

Individuals with cancer are more susceptible to infection for a number of reasons. Tumours themselves may damage the protective barriers of skin or membranes [19,20)], or obstruct a bronchus or ureter [21]. Brain tumours may interfere with control of bladder emptying or lead to loss of the gag reflex, leading to aspiration pneumonia. Some cancers, particularly myeloma and chronic lymphocytic leukaemia - directly interfere with humoral immunity [22]. Some leukaemias - chronic lymphocytic leukaemia, for example, cause hypogammaglobulinaemia, which leads to bacterial infections of the respiratory, urinary tracts and skin, often with *Strep.pneumoniae* or coliforms [23]. Cell mediated immunity and phagocytosis may be compromised either by malignancy or the chemotherapy used to treat it. Splenectomy makes individuals highly susceptible to *Strep.pneumoniae* and other species of bacteria [19]. Infected Hickman lines will be only too familiar to any physician who has worked on an oncology ward [24]. The flora that tend to colonise debilitated individuals are more likely to be pathogenic [25].

Neutropaenia or pancytopaenia are predictable sequelae of chemotherapy. The febrile neutropaenic patient requires swift attention. Empirical therapy may need to be started before cultures are available or other diagnostic procedures embarked upon or results obtained to prevent threatening sepsis. An important principle is that with successive episodes of neutropaenia the organisms causing infection will be different. Gut flora will have altered after exposure to antibiotics. There will also have been a longer acquaintance with hospital commensals and environmental agents such as *Aspergillus.*

In malignancy latent viruses, particularly *herpes simplex,* may reactivate [26]; open ulcers in skin or mucosa then allow secondary infections such as *Candida* or *Aspergillus* to occur [27]. Paradoxically, with the improvement in survival for many cancers, infections are likely to prove increasingly common in this group.

Post Surgery

The successful management of peri-operative sepsis has allowed modern surgery to develop. Infections remain common, and may occur in 3-4% of surgical wounds [28,29]. The likelihood of wound infection depends on the immune status of the host; the size and site of the wound, local trauma, including haematoma and devitalization of tissues, the nature of the invading organism and its exposure to prophylactic antibiotics, and the degree of sterility of the procedure. Respiratory and urinary tract infections are common due to immobility. Blood transfusion increases the risk of infection [30].

The febrile, unwell post-operative patient is a frequent clinical problem, and diagnosis is not always easy. Deeper abscesses may demand radiological investigation. Furthermore, non-infective causes of fever such as DVT, PE and drug or transfusion reactions must also be considered.

Nosocomial Infections

Nosocomial infection accounts for a large proportion of morbidity in hospital patients. Infections of the chest are especially important, and up to 15% of all deaths in hospitals may be due to hospital-acquired pneumonia [31]. Urinary tract infections are the commonest of any type of infection in hospitals and nursing homes, and most are catheter related [32]. Intensive care units and recovery rooms are particularly vulnerable, because these individuals are already unwell or unconscious and the presentation may not be classical. Fever, cough, sputum or chest X-ray changes might not occur or may be due to non-infective causes. It might be difficult therefore to decide whether a microbiological isolate is infecting the lung or airways or merely colonising them. The tendency however is to underdiagnose [34][33].

Multiple Trauma

Advances in the management of severe trauma have improved survival in this group. Infection is now more important as a cause of morbidity and mortality. Of those who survive their injuries, approximately one half of subsequent deaths are due to infection [34]. Contamination, ischaemia, intubation, protheses, drains, catheters and the problems attendent on immobility and hospitalization all contribute to a greater incidence of infection [35]. There is also ample evidence of defective immunity and phagocytosis in the traumatized patient [36,37].

There are problems in the diagnosis of infection in these individuals. The patient may be artificially ventilated, covered in bandages, unconscious, confused or in too much pain for thorough examination and too haemodynamically unstable for radiological assessment. The conventional signs of infection-fever, leucocytosis and tachycardia, may be related to the injury, haematoma or other non-infectious causes. Drug and alcohol withdrawal are common in accident and burn victims and may mimic infection [38].

Burns

The greater the surface area affected by burns, the greater the chance of infection and subsequent mortality [39]. The causes of infection following burns are complex, and relate to several factors including the presence of dead tissue and to depression of cellular and humoral immune function. Deranged neutrophil function also seems to be the major determinant [40,41], although the mechanisms surrounding this process are unclear.

A major difficulty in the management of burn wound infections lies in deciding when bacterial colonization has become pathogenic. Cultures do not afford the answer, although clinical signs will often be very suggestive, and the only reliable investigation is biopsy [42]. Pneumonia may also occur after, as a consequence of smoke inhalation or result from other factors associated with large surface-area burns [43]. Septic thrombophlebitis is a complication which carries a high mortality and is difficult to diagnose [44]. Bacterial endocarditis may also occur [45]. Electrical burns sometimes cause deeper tissue necrosis and abscesses [46] with relatively little visible surface damage.

Spinal Cord Injury

Infections frequently arise following damage to the spinal cord and pneumonia is the leading cause of death, particularly when patients are ventilated [47]. Aspiration is common particularly, with higher cord lesions. Bladder emptying is often defective making urinary tract infection (UTI) more likely, especially in the elderly [48]. UTI is almost inevitable in people with SCI who have indwelling or intermittent catheterisation [49]. Immobility tends to lead to pressure sores, which may become contaminated by faeces and urine [50], and osteomyelitis may supervene. All of these conditions may lead to bacteraemia [51]. Occasionally the problem arises of a paralysed patient with recurrent bacteraemia with no obvious source. The cause is often found to be an occult abscess [52]. Elevated levels of acute phase proteins in these patients may suggest underlying infection is undiagnosed. Occasionally deranged autonomic control causes spontaneous self-limiting fevers without infection [53], and rarely this may be prolonged.

Transplant Recipients

Transplantation of major organs is being performed increasingly frequently. There are many reasons why the transplant recipient is at increased risk of infection. The risk of severe infections is greatest in the weeks and months following the transplant, and after six months mortality from infection falls [54,55]. The majority of symptomatic infections are bacterial and relate to surgery (intra-abdominal, biliary and wound infections), ventilation and indwelling intravenous cannulae [56]. The high incidence of early infection may be explained by a number of factors. Individuals may still be suffering from the condition which provoked the need for transplant, or other medical conditions [57]. The stress of surgery also diminishes host resistance, and there is the risk of exposure to hospital acquired infections to which the patient may not have protective immunity. Local infection at the operation site or via a Hickman line is common [24]. Latent infection may reactivate, for example tuberculosis and *herpes simplex* [58].

Immunosuppressive drugs are usually prescribed. Infection with some agents, for example cytomegalovirus (CMV), make further superinfections more likely. CMV also appears to promote changes within the allograft that increase the risk of chronic rejection [59]. Graft versus host disease (GVHD) and host versus graft disease may also predispose to infection, often with opportunists such as aspergillosis and CMV pneumonitis. Chronic GVHD may lead to reactivation of herpes zoster which in this setting may be widespread and even fatal.

Fever amongst transplant recipients is common. Immunosuppressive drugs may suppress fever but fortunately in practice this is rare. The source of sepsis is often obvious, but fever of unknown origin with negative blood cultures is a frequent finding. CMV is a common cause, but the differential diagnosis should include deep abscesses, candidiasis, toxoplasmosis and oneumocytosis. Rejection, drug reactions, thrombotic disease and infarction are other common causes of fever in this situation.

HIV

Pulmonary infection is a major cause of illness in patients with the Human Immunodeficiency Virus (HIV) [60]. Tuberculous lung disease is of increasing concern. Multiple drug resistant tuberculosis, defined as resistance to two or more of the drugs commonly used to treat the disease, has occurred as outbreaks in the USA, UK and elsewhere. Diagnostic difficulties do arise in the AIDS patient with respiratory symptoms. Induced sputum examination has limited positive and negative predictive value, and bronchoalveolar lavage often has to be performed, with or without transbronchial biopsy. Open lung biopsy may have to be resorted to where the above are unhelpful or there is coagulopathy. A major difficulty lies in differentiating pulmonary Kaposi's sarcoma from other causes of breathlessness, unproductive cough and sometimes fever [61]. It is largely a diagnosis of exclusion, although bronchoscopy, gallium scans and transbronchial biopsy may yield useful information.

The gastrointestinal tract can be affected by a range of pathogenic processes in AIDS. Where in most cases diagnosis may be established by endoscopy, biopsy and culture, difficulties do arise with a number of clinical presentations. The patient with right upper quadrant pain and tenderness, fever and an elevated alkaline phosphatase is one of these. Acalculous cholangitis, possibly associated with cryptosporidium or cytomegalovirus, sclerosing cholangitis and papillary stenosis are all differential diagnoses [62].

Another example is the AIDS patient with persistent diarrhoea and negative stool cultures, with negative upper and lower GI endoscopy and biopsy. Between 15 and 20% of patients with persistent diarrhoea fall into this group. AIDS-associated enteropathy is said to be the cause, although much of this probably due to a number of pathogens yet to be identified. Clostridium difficile associated pseudomembranous colitis is a common complication in in-patients with AIDS [63].

Diagnostic difficulties arise in categorising intracranial mass lesions in HIV (table 1). They tend do arise late in disease and symptoms may be non-specific and even unimpressive. Even histopathological examination of biopsy or post-mortem specimens fails to provide a diagnosis in approximately 10%. Toxoplasmosis is the most frequent cause, followed by lymphoma, progressive multifocal leucoencephalopathy (PML), tuberculosis and other agents listed elsewhere. Radiology is often helpful but rarely pathognomonic. Clinical features may help in choosing empirical treatment for the likeliest cause, e.g. *Toxoplasma gondii*. Definitive diagnosis may require CSF examination and culture or brain biopsy. This investigation may be considered where progressive multifocal leucoencephalopathy is suspected. This demyelinating disease of cerebral white matter is associated with the eponymous JC and BK papovaviruses [64]. It commonly presents with headache, ataxia, hemiparesis and other mental state changes. It may be seen on MRI as high intensity lesions that do not enhance. Diagnostic difficulty may arise with Cryptococcal meningitis. Once again, symptoms may be vague and there may only be a low grade fever and possibly headache. Confirmation of the diagnosis is made by staining CSF with Indian Ink, CSF culture, and by testing for cryptococcal antigen in serum and CSF.

HIV can directly infect the meninges and brain substance. There may be an acute or relapsing meningitis, although this may be asymptomatic despite evidence of HIV in the CSF [65]. The syndrome of AIDS dementia complex occurs in 15-20% of individuals with more advanced disease. Imaging of the brain, particularly by CT scanning or MRI, shows cerebral atrophy not consistent with the patient's age.

The other central nervous organ susceptible to opportunist infection in AIDS is the eye. Up to 60% of AIDS patients will develop Cytomegalovirus retinitis, leading to progressive painless visual loss. ***Varicella zoster [66], toxoplasma gondii*** and ***pneumocystis carinii*** [67] may also cause retinitis.

Polymyositis, pyomyositis and rheumatological disorders occur in patients with AIDS for a number of causes related to HIV and other infective agents, such as gonococcus, septic arthritis, hepatitis B and Reiter's disease. The diagnostic difficulty lies in establishing which is the most likely cause.

The skin of the AIDS patient is prone to infection with certain viruses, particularly the herpes and pox groups, and opportunistic bacterial and fungal agents. A newly described syndrome of bacillary angiomatosis is attributed to the organisms of ***Bartonella*** spp. The skin lesions may disseminate and cause a characteristic illness known as bacillary peliosis presenting as right upper quadrant pain, hepatomegaly and elevated alkaline phosphatase [68]. Diagnosis is by biopsy, and must be differentiated from other causes of the same presentation outlined above.

Table 1. Space Occupying CNS Lesions in AIDS

    a] Malignancies

        Lymphoma, primary and secondary

        Kaposi's Sarcoma

    b] Infections

        Tuberculosis

        Toxoplasmosis

        Cryptococcosis

        Nocardiosis

        Histoplasmosis

        Cytomegalovirus

        Herpes Simplex

        HIV

        Candidiasis

        Progressive Multifocal Leucoencephalopathy (JC/BK virus)

The challenge with renal impairment in AIDS lies in differentiating HIV-associated nephropathy from other causes [69]. Drugs, IVDA, hepatitis B, hypertension and malignancies may all complicate the issue. True HIV-related nephropathy tends to occur late in the disease and responds poorly to haemodialysis.

Intravenous Drug Abusers [IVDA]

Management of this group of patients is compounded by social and behavioural circumstances. Intravenous drug abuse is a risk factor for the acquisition of HIV, and this increases the risk of multiple simultaneous infections. The increased incidence of viral hepatitis is well described [70]. Infection with resistant organisms such as multi resistant **Staphylococcus Aureus** is common, as drug abusers may have open skin infections which are sites for colonisation. They may also self treat with antibiotics [71]. This also means that bacterial cultures may be falsely negative.

Although the emphasis has been on bacterial endocarditis the commonest infections are of the skin and soft tissues [72]. Repeated injection of unsterilized and contaminated material is the obvious source. These skin infections may lead to septicaemia and death. HIV infected individuals are prone to   precisely the same organisms, predominantly **Staphylococcus Aureaus** and **Streptococcus,** particularly **Milleri.** Mouth organisms are common as substances may be crushed between the teeth before injection [73], or the injection site may be "cleaned" with saliva or the needle licked. Deep abscesses may result which can be difficult to diagnose, whereas superficial cellulitis is readily visible. Abusers may switch injection sites as their veins trombose, and abscesses may occur in any site, including the neck, mediastinum and groin, sometimes with catastrophic consequences as erosion or compression involves local structures [74]. An important complication that is difficult to confirm is osteomyelitis [75]. There is often a periosteal reaction in uninfected bones underlying large ulcers, and a bone scan or even biopsy may be required. Infections of bones and joints by haematogenous seeding may also occur and is difficult to diagnose [72]. There may be few symptoms or signs or little radiological evidence. A wide range of organisms may responsible, including mycobacteria and fungi.

Abscesses, pseudo- and myotic aneurysms also occur in peripheral blood vessels, usually by local infection. Necrotising fasciitis may arise in drug abusers [76] and the classic signs are often absent; the appearance may be of a simple cellulitis. The only clue may be that pain and systemic upset are out of proportion to the extent of the apparent infection. Bullae, crepitus, high fever and necrosis of the skin may not develop until later, by which time serious morbidity or mortality is likely.

Symptoms and signs of bacterial endocarditis may not be classical. Osler's nodes and other stigmata are rare. The patient may present with general systemic upset or dyspnoea from emboli in right sided infections. The most sensitive test is culture of the blood, which is positive in 80-100% [77]. Vegetations are found on echocardiography in up to 94% [78]. Local and peripheral abscesses may arise. Splenic abscesses may complicate endocarditis, or arise separately [79,80]. Bacterial endocarditis tends to recur in IVDAs, and while it is normal to survive the first episode the prognosis is poor if addiction persists. The 10 year survival may be as low as 10% [81].

The differential diagnosis in the febrile IVDA with an abnormal CXR must include infectious and non-infectious. There is an increase in community acquired pneumonias [82].

Septic emboli and pulmonary infarcts may be indistinguishable from pneumonia. Lung abscesses may arise, as may tuberculosis [83]. There are also the opportunistic lung infections caused by AIDS to consider [60].

Non infectious causes of damage to the lungs in IVDA include opiate induced pulmonary oedema, or drug associated asthma [84]. Talc, used as a bulking agent [85], may cause granulomatosis. Aspiration is also more common.

Either drugs or infection are common causes of neurological disease in IVDAs and both may cause coma, encephalopathy, confusion, seizures, Parkinsonism and dementia. Septic and mycotic emboli arise most often from endocarditis, and may cause brain abscesses, endophthalmitis or meningitis. Spinal abscess with cord compression may develop. Tetanus and botulism are also slightly more common, although the incidence of the former is falling in IVDA [86].

Between 5 and 10% of IVDAs worldwide are infected with HIV, with a figure as high as 60% in some studies [82]. This condition is discussed above. Other sexually transmitted diseases are also more common in IVDA, and this is partly due to a high incidence of prostitution [87].

FUO

The definition of FUO or PUO [88] has lately been revised, although it has not achieved WHO classification. FUO can usefully be subdivided into classic, nosocomial, neutripaenic and HIV-associated [89]. The original definition [88] required an illness of more than three weeks with documented fevers above 38.3° on separate occasions with no diagnosis after one week as an in-patient. Exceptions to these criteria exist, e.g. in neutropaenic FUO the duration of negative investigation is reduced to three days.

FUO requires a systematic approach. More thans 70% of individuals will have one of three causes-infection, malignancy or autoimmune disease [90]. Tuberculosis (42%), visceral leishmaniasis (14%), and disseminated Myobacterium avium complex infection (14%) were the most frequent diagnosis. In HIV-associated FUO in one study [91], but the causes depend on the infections endemic in the particular region. Other diagnoses include granulomatous, thrombo-embolic and drug-related disorders. Diagnostic laparotomy is still occasionally required [92], but with improved non-invasive imaging and diagnostic techniques this is becoming increasingly unusual. A growing proportion of patients with FUO elude definitive diagnosis [93] even after prolonged follow-up and re-evaluation [94]. There is a further small group of individuals with exaggerated circadian temperature rhythm. In both of these two groups, the prognosis is excellent.

Zoonoses

There are well over 150 zoonotic diseases described so far. Some zoonoses are extremely common. Cryptosporidiosis, for example, has a seroprevalence of up to 35% and 64% in the developed and third world respectively [95]. Zoonoses may be severe and epidemic, for example, the great plagues of history, of which the recent outbreak in India was a less severe example [96], or rabies, which kills between 30 and 50.000 people each year in India alone [97].

The main reason for late diagnosis of a zoonosis is a low index of suspicion. The best clue usually lies in the history. The diagnosis of leptospirosis in a jaundiced sewage worker may be obvious, but less obvious examples of exposure to domestic animals or transient exposure to farmyard or wild animals are often missed [98]. Diagnosis is usually confirmed by serology or culture.

Tropical Travellers

The unwell returning is an increasingly problem. The speed of modern international travel has meant that individuals may return home long before the incubation of their illness is complete. Some infections - hepatitides, schistosomiasis and malaria, for example, may only develop months or even years after leaving the endemic area, and they may be unaware of the possible exposure [99].

In one study [100], malaria headed the list of diagnosis of the febrile traveller returning from the tropics. Other illnesses are listed in table 1. A number of avoidable deaths occur each year due to delay in the diagnosis of malaria [101]. Intestinal helminths are also common. In a proportion of returning febrile travellers a diagnosis is never made [see table 2].

Table 2. *Aetiology of fever after travel to tropics. Values are percentages of patients. From [102] with kind permission of the author.*

Diagnosis	Maclean *et al* [103] [n=587]	Doherty *et al* [100] [n=195]
Malaria	32	42
Hepatitis	6	3
Respiratory infection*	11	2.5
Urinary Tract infection	4	2.5
Dengue fever	2	6
Enteric fever	2	2
Diarrhoeal illness	4.5	6.5
Epstein-Barr virus	2	0.5
Pharyngitis	1	2
Rickettsia	1	0.5
Amoebic liver abscess	1	0
Tuberculosis	1	2
Meningitis	1	1
Acute HIV infection	0.3	1
Miscellaneous	6.3	5
Undiagnosed	25	24.5†

*Includes upper respiratory tract infection, bronchitis, and pneumonia.

†Includes presumed viral and non-specific infections.

References

1. Lichtman SM. Physiological aspects of aging. Implications for the treatment of cancer. Drugs Aging [1995];7[3]: 212-25.
2. Norman DC, Toledo SD. Infections in elderly persons. An altered clinical presentation. [Review]. Clin Geriatric Med [1992];8(4): 713-9.
3. Evans JG. General medicine and geriatrics, where is the difference? The example of infective disease. Schweiz Med Wochenschr [1995];125[40]: 1847-54.
4. Saltzman RL, Peterson PK. Immunodeficiency of the elderly. [Review]. Reviews of Infectious Diseases [1987];9[6]: 1127-39.
5. Ben YA, Weksler ME. Host resistance and the immune system. [Review]. Clin Geriatric Med [1992];8[4]: 701-11.
6. Rummans TA, Evans JM, Krahn LE, Fleming KC. Delirium in elderly patients: evaluation and management. Mayo Clin Proc [1995];70[10]: 989-98.
7. Melchior H. [Disorders of bladder function in the elderly]. Urologe A [1995];34[4]: 329-33.
8. Lew J, Glass R, Gangarosa R, et al. Diarrheal deaths in the United States, 1979 through 1987. JAMA [1991];265: 3280-4.
9. Woodhead M. Pneumonia in the elderly. J Antimicrob Chemother [1994];
10. Bentley DW. Bacterial pneumonia in the elderly: clinical features, diagnosis, etiology, and treatment. [Review]. Gerontology [1984];30[5]: 297-307.
11. Heuser MD, Case LD, Ettinger WH. Mortality in intensive care patients with respiratory disease. Is age important? Arch Intern Med [1992];152[8]: 1683-8.
12. Yoshikawa TT, Norman DC. Infection control in long-term care. Clin Geriatr Med [1995];11[3]: 467-80.
13. Leibovici L. Bacteraemia in the very old. Features and treatment. Drugs Aging [1995];6[6]: 456-64.
14. Gransden WR, Eykyn SJ, Phillips I. Septicaemia in the newborn and elderly. J Antimicrob Chemother [1994];
15. Meyers BR, Sherman E, Mendelson MH, et al. Bloodstream infections in the elderly [see comments]. Am J Med [1989];86[4]: 379-84.
16. Richardson JP. Bacteremia in the elderly. [Review]. J Gen Intern Med [1993];8[2]: 89-92.
17. Matthews D. The prevention and diagnosis of infective endocarditis. The primary care provider's role. Nurse Pract [1994];19[8]: 53-60.
18. Norman DC, Yoshikawa TT. Infections of the bone, joint, and bursa. Clin Geriatr Med [1994];10[4]: 703-18.
19. Rosenberg AS, Brown AE. Infection in the cancer patient. [Review]. Disease A Month [1993];39[7]: 505-69.
20. Krishnasamy M. Oral problems in advanced cancer. Eur J Cancer Care Engl [1995];4[4]: 173-7.
21. Casey KR. Neoplastic mimics of pneumonia. Semin Respir Infect [1995];10[3]: 131-42.
22. Binet I, Schifferli JA. [Infectious risk factors with special attention to elderly patients.] Schweiz Med Wochenschr [1994];124[49]: 2226-8.
23. Das PK, Chhotaray MK, Rath RN, Kar S, Das B, Parida B. Infection in haematological malignancies. J Indian Med Assoc [1994];92[10]: 328-30.
24. Farr BM. Vascular catheter related infections in cancer patients. Surg Oncol Clin N Am [1995];4[3]: 493-503.
25. Immunosuppressive drugs and their complications. Drug Ther Bull [1994];32[9]: 66-70.
26. Devine SM, Wingard JR. Viral infections in severely immunocompromised cancer patients. Support Care Cancer [1994];2[6]: 355-68.

27. Benedict S, Colagreco J. Fungal infections associated with malignancies, treatments, and AIDS. Cancer Nurs [1994];**17**[5]: 411-7.

28. Wenzel RP. Preoperative antibiotic prophylaxis [editorial; comment]. N Engl J Med [1992];**326** [5]: 337-9.

29. Haley RW, Culver DH, White JW, Morgan WM, Emori TG. The nationwide nosocomial infection rate. A new need for vital statistics. Am J Epidemiol [1985];**121**[2]: 159-67.

30. Cafiero F, Gipponi M, Bonalumi U, Piccardo A, Sguotti C, Corbetta G. Prophylaxis of infection with intravenous immunoglobulins plus antibiotic for patients at risk for sepsis undergoing surgery for colorectal cancer: results of a randomized, multicenter clinical trial. Surgery [1992];**112**[1]: 24-31.

31. Salemi C, Morgan J, Padilla S, Morissey R. Association between severity of illness and mortality from nosocomial infection. Am J Infect Control [1995];**23**[3]: 188-93.

32. Colling J, McCreedy M, Owen T. Urinary tract infection rates among incontinent nursing home and community dwelling elderly. Urol Nurs [1994];**14**[3]: 117-9.

33. Andrews CP, Coalson JJ, Smith JD, Johanson WJ. Diagnosis of nosocomial bacterial pneumonia in acute, diffuse lung injury. Chest [1981];**80**[3]: 254-8.

34. Bassin AS, Niederman MS. New approaches to prevention and treatment of nosocomial pneumonia. Semin Thorac Cardiovasc Surg [1995];**7**[2]: 70-7.

35. Von RK, Harris JR. Pulmonary dysfunction related to immobility in the trauma patient. Aacn Clin Issues [1995];**6**[2]: 212-28.

36. Napolitano LM, Campbell C. Polymicrobial sepsis following trauma inhibits interleukin-10 secretion and lymphocyte proliferation. J Trauma [1995];**39**[1]: 104-10.

37. O'Sullivan ST, Lederer JA, Horgan AF, Chin DH, Mannick JA, Rodrick ML. Major injury leads to predominance of the T helper-2 lymphocyte phenotype and diminished interleukin-12 production associated with decreased resistance to infection. Ann Surg [1995];**222**[4]: 482-90.

38. Haum A, Perbix W, Hack HJ, Stark GB, Spilker G, Doehn M. Alcohol and drug abuse in burn injuries. Burns [1995];**21**[3]: 194-9.

39. Ward RS, Saffle JR. Topical agents in burn and wound care. Phys Ther [1995];**75**[6]: 526-38.

40. Griswold JA. White blood cell response to burn injury. Semin Nephrol [1993];**13**[4]: 409-15.

41. Heideman M, Bengtsson A. The immunologic response to thermal injury. World J Surg [1992];**16**[1]: 53-6.

42. Pruitt BJ, McManus AT. The changing epidemiology of infection in burn patients. World J Surg [1992];**16**[1]: 57-67.

43. Nguyen TT, Gilpin DA, Meyer NA, Herndon DN. Current treatment of severely burned patients. Ann Surg [1996];**223**[1]: 14-25.

44. Levine NS, Salisbury RE. Infection in the burned upper extremity. Major Problems Clin Surg [1976];**19**[47]: 47-62.

45. Winkelman MD, Galloway PG. Central nervous system complications of thermal burns. A postmortem study of 139 patients. Medicine [1992];**71**[5]: 271-83.

46. Yakuboff KP, Kurtzman LC, Stern PJ. Acute management of thermal and electrical burns of the upper extremity. [Review.] Orth Clin N Am [1992];**23**[1]: 161-9.

47. DeVivo MJ, Ivie C3. Life expectancy of ventilator-dependent persons with spinal cord injuries. Chest [1995];**108**[1]: 226-32.

48. Komura T, Yamasaki M, Muraki S, Seki K. Characteristics of the health conditions of old patients with spinal cord injury. J Hem Ergol Tokyo [1994];**23**[2]: 151-7.

49. Cardenas DD, Hooton TM. Urinary tract infection in persons with spinal cord injury. Arch Phys Med Rehab [1995];**76**[3]: 272-80.

50. Hammond MC, Bozzacco VA, Stiens SA, Buhrer R, Lyman P. Pressure ulcer incidence on a spinal cord injury unit. Adv Wound Care [1994];**7**[6]: 57-60.

51. McBride DQ, Rodts GE. Intensive care of patients with spinal trauma. Neurosurg Clin N Am

[1994];**5**[4]: 755-66.

52. Jang TN, Fung CP. Treatment of pyogenic splenic abscess: nonsurgical procedures. J Formos Med Assoc [1995];**94**[6]: 309-12.

53. Colachis S, Otis SM. Occurrence of fever associated with thermoregulatory dysfunction after acute traumatic spinal cord injury. Am J Phys Med Rehab [1995];**74**[2]: 114-9.

54. Shaw BJ, Martin DJ, Marquez JM, et al. Venous bypass in clinical liver transplantation. Ann Surg [1984];**200**[4]: 524-34.

55. Starzl TE, Klintmalm GB, Porter KA, Iwatsuki S, Schroter GP. Liver transplantation with use of cyclosporin a and prednisone. N Engl J Med [1981];**305**[5]: 266-9.

56. Kibbler CC. Infections in liver transplantations: risk factors and strategies for prevention. J Hosp Infect [1995];

57. Tolkoff RN, Rubin RH. The infectious disease problems of the diabetic renal transplant recipient. Infect Dis Clin North Am [1995];**9**[1]: 117-30.

58. Avery RK, Longworth DL. Viral pulmonary infections in thoracic and cardiovascular surgery. Semin Thorac Cardiovasc Surg [1995];**7**[2]: 88-94.

59. Keenan RJ, Zeevi A. Immunologic consequences of transplantation. Chest Surg Clin N Am [1995];**5**[1]: 107-20.

60. Mitchell DM, Miller RF. AIDS and the lung: update 1995. 2. New developments in the pulmonary diseases affecting HIV infected individuals. [Review]. Thorax [1995];**50**[3]: 294-302.

61. Garay SM, Belenko M, Fazzini E, Schinella R. Pulmonary manifestations of Kaposi's sarcoma. Chest [1987];**91**[1]: 39-43.

62. Margulis S, Honig C, Soave R, et al. Biliary tract obstruction in the acquired immunodeficiency syndrome. Ann Intern Med [1986];**105**: 207.

63. Peters B, Carlin E, Weston R, Loveless S, Sweney J, Weber J, Main J. Adverse effects of drugs used in the management of opportunistic infections associated with HIV infection. Drug Safety [1994];[10]: 439-454.

64. Chaisson RE, Griffin DE. Progressive multifocal leucoencephalopathy in AIDS [clinical conference]. JAMA [1990];**264**[1]: 79-82.

65. Hollander H, Stringari S. Human immunodeficiency virus-associated meningitis. Clinical course and correlations. Am J Med [1987];**83**[5]: 813-6.

66. Margolis TP, Lowder CY, Holland GN, et al. Varicella-zoster virus retinitis in patients with the acquired immunodeficiency syndrome. Am J Ophthalmol [1991];**112**[2]: 119-31.

67. Wasserman L, Haghighi P. Optic and ophthalmic pneumocystosis in acquired immunodeficiency syndrome. Report of a case and review of the literature. [Review]. Arch Pathol Lab Med [1992];**116** [5]: 500-3.

68. Koehler J, LeBoit P, Egbert B, et al. Cutaneous vascular lesions and disseminated cat-scratch disease in patients with AIDS and AIDS-related complex. Ann Intern Med [1988];**109**: 449-55.

69. Rao TK, Filippone EJ, Nicastri AD, et al. Associated focal and segmental glomerulosclerosis in the acquired immunodeficiency syndrome. N Engl J Med [1984];**310**[11]: 669-73.

70. Eber B, Rabenau H, Berger A, et al. Seroprevalence of HCV, HAV, HBV, HDV, HCMV and HIV in high risk groups/Frankfurt a.M., Germany. Int J Med Microbiol Virol Parasitol Infect Dis [1995];**282**[1]: 102-12.

71. Crane LR, Levine DP, Zervos MJ, Commings G. Bacteremia in narcotic addicts at the Detroit Medical Center. I. Microbiology, epidemiology, risk factors and empiric therapy. Rev Infect Dis [1986];**8**[3]: 364-73.

72. Henriksen BM, Albrektsen SB, Simper LB, Gutschik E. Soft tissue infections from drug abuse. A clinical and microbiological review of 145 cases. Acta Orthop Scand [1994];**65**[6]: 625-8.

73. Hemingway DM, Balfour AE, McCartney AC, Leiberman DP. Streptococcus milleri and complex groin abscesses in intravenous drug abusers. Scottish Med J [1992];**37**[4]: 116-7.

74. Wallace JR, Lucas CE, Ledgerwood AM. Social, economic, and surgical anatomy of a drug-related abscess. Am Surgeon [1986];**52**[7]: 398-401.

75. Wald ER. Risk factors for osteomyelitis. [Review]. Am J Med [1985];**78**[6B]: 206-12.

76. Bosch U. [Compartment syndrome of the pelvis]. [German]. Unfallchirurg [1991];**94**[5]: 244-8.

77. Komshian SV, Tablan OC, Palutke W, Reyes MP. Characteristics of left-sided endocarditis due to Pseudomonas aeruginosa in the Detroit Medical Center. Rev Infect Dis [1990];**12**[4]: 693-702.

78. Weisse AB, Heller DR, Schimenti RJ, Montgomery RL, Kapila R. The febrile parenteral drug user: a prospective study in 121 patients. Am J Med [1993];**94**[3]: 274-80.

79. Nallathambi MN, Ivatury RR, Lankin DH, Wapnir IL, Stahl WM. Pyogenic splenic abscess in intravenous drug addiction. Am Surgeon [1987];**53**[6]: 342-6.

80. Fry DE, Richardson JD, Flint LM. Occult splenic abscess: an unrecognized complication of heroin abuse. Surgery [1978];**84**[5]: 650-4.

81. Frater RW. Surgical management of endocarditis in drug addicts and long-term results. J Cardiac Surg [1990];**5**[1]: 63-7.

82. O'Donnell AE, Selig J, Aravamuthan M, Richardson MS. Pulmonary complications associated with illicit drug use. Chest [1995];**108**[2]: 460-3.

83. Brown LJ, Hickson MJ, Ajuluchukwu DC, Bailey J. Medical disorders in a cohort of New York city drug abusers: much more than HIV disease. J Addict Dis [1993];**12**[4]: 11-27.

84. Perper JA, Van TD. Respiratory complications of cocaine abuse. Recent Dev Alcohol [1992];**10**[363]: 363-77.

85. Sherman KE, Lewey SM, Goodman ZD. Talc in the liver of patients with chronic hepatitis C infection. Am J Gastroenterol [1995];**90**[12]: 2164-6.

86. Cherubin CE, Sapira JD. The medical complications of drug addiction and the medical assessment of the intravenous drug user: 25 years later [see comments]. Ann Intern Med [1993];**119**[10]: 1017-28.

87. Fortenberry JD. Adolescent substance use and sexually transmitted disease risk: a review. J Adolesc Health [1995];**16**[4]: 304-8.

88. Petersdorf R, Beeson P. Fever of unexplained origin: Report of 100 cases. Medicine [1961];**40**: 1.

89. Durack D, Street A. Fever of unknown origin - re-examined and redefined. In: Remington J, Swartz M, ed. Current Clinical Topics of Infectious Diseases. St. Louis, Mo: Mosby-Year Book, Inc, 1991: 35.

90. Wong SY, Lam MS. Pyrexia of unknown origin-approach to management. Singapore Med J [1995];**36**[2]: 204-8.

91. Miralles P, Moreno S, Perez TM, Cosin J, Diaz MD, Bouza E. Fever of uncertain origin in patients infected with the human immunodeficiency virus. Clin Infect Dis [1995];**20**[4]: 872-5.

92. Rothman DL, Schwartz SI, Adams JT. Diagnostic laparotomy for fever or abdominal pain of unknown origin. Am J Surg [1977];**133**[3]: 273-5.

93. de Kleijn E, van der Meer J. Fever of unknown origin (FUO): report on 53 patients in a Dutch university hospital. Neth J Med [1995];**47**[2]: 54-60.

94. Knockaert DC, Vanneste LJ, Vanneste SB, Bobbaers HJ. Fever of unknown origin in the 1980s. An update of the diagnostic spectrum. Arch Intern Med [1992];**152**[1]: 51-5.

95. Navin TR, Juranek DD. Cryptosporidiosis: clinical, epidemiologic, and parasitologic review. [Review]. Rev Infect Dis [1984];**6**[3]: 313-27.

96. Gushulak BD, St JR, Jeychandran T, Coksedge W. Human plague in India, August-October, 1994. Can Commun Dis Rep [1994];**20**[20]: 181-3.

97. Warrell DA, Warrell MJ. Human rabies: a continuing challenge in the tropical world. Schweiz Med Wochenschr [1995];**125**[18]: 879-85.

98. Langley JM, Marrie TJ, Covert A, Waag DM, Williams JC. Poker players' pneumonia. An urban outbreak of Q fever following exposure to a parturient cat. N Engl J Med [1988];**319**[6]: 354-6.

99. Wolfe MS. Diseases of travellers. Clin Symposia [1984];**36**[2]: 2-32.

100. Doherty JF, Grant AD, Bryceson AD. Fever as the presenting complaint of travellers returning from the tropics. QJM [1995];**88**[4]: 277-81.

101. Bradley D, Warhurst D, Blaze M, Smith V. Malaria imported into the United Kingdom in 1992 and 1993. Commun Dis Reo Cdr Rev [1994];**4**[1]):
102. Humar A, Keystone J. Evaluating fevers in travellers returning from tropical countries. Br Med J [1996];**312**[7036]: 953-956.
103. Maclean J, Lalonde R, Ward B. Fever from the tropics. In: Travel Medicine Advisor. 1994: 27.1-27.14 vol 5.

CHAPTER 2

RADIOPHARMACEUTICALS FOR IMAGING INFECTIOUS AND
INFLAMMATORY FOCI

Peter H. Cox

Introduction

It is well known that a number of radiopharmaceuticals show a non specific uptake in
inflammatory processes. Whilst this may be of some diagnostic value there is a need for
reagents which localise specifically in foci of inflammation and which distinguish between
infection and aseptic inflammatory processes not to mention occult foci of infection and
non specific tumour uptake. Such a requirement immediately introduces the concept that
different classes of radiopharmaceutical will be required to distinguish these types of lesion
from one another. Inflammatory foci do not have a specific receptor to which a potential
radiopharmaceutical can be targeted but whilst the inflammatory process is a complicated
phenomenon it does have a number of features which can positively influence the
accumulation of radiopharmaceuticals in the lesion.

These include erythema accompanied by an increased permeability of the walls of the small
blood vessels. This in turn leads to oedema due to leakage blood components into the
interstitial space. At the same time there is a parallel migration of leucocytes into the
inflamed area. Chemical mediators are released including chemotactic substances which
attract and activate phagocytic cells. The cell membrane permeability of normal tissue may
increase and indeed lysis may occur. These phenomena may be seen as mechanisms
whereby a radiopharmaceutical can become deposited in a focus of inflammation in higher
concentrations than in normal tissue. Medium to high molecular weight proteins, synthetic
polymers and particulate colloids are able to pass through the fenestrations in the arterioles
and capillaries to collect in oedema fluid, particulate colloids may also be ingested by
phagocytes and the latter can also be targeted by radiolabelled antigranulocyte antibodies.
Leucocytes can also be labelled by various other methods so that they themselves function
as ligands. Ionic metal complexes also localise non specifically in foci of inflammation
partly intracellularly and partly in oedema fluid whilst labelled antibiotics may show a

21

P. H.Cox and J. R. Buscombe (eds.), The Imaging of Infection and Inflammation, 21-29.
© 1998 *Kluwer Academic Publishers. Printed in the Netherlands.*

preference for infection foci. Clearly with all of these factors influencing radiopharmaceutical uptake the physiological status of the lesion will determine the success rate of a given radiopharmaceutical. Although several factors may play a role in the localisation of a radiopharmaceutical it is convenient to classify them according to the prime mechanism which influences their uptake [figure 1].

```
Non specific reagents localising in Oedema:
     Technetium-99m HIg.
     Technetium Hydrazinonicotinamide IgG.
     Indium-111 IgM.
     Indium-111 IgG.
     Technetium-99m Nanocolloid.
     Technetium-99m MPEG-PL-DTPA [synthetic polymer]

Non Specific reagents showing local phagocyte uptake:
     Gallium-67 Citrate.
     Indium-111 Chloride.
     Technetium-99m Nanocolloid.
     Indium-111 Liposomes
     Technetium-99m "stealth" Liposomes

Antibody:
     Indium-111 Fab'₂ 1.2B6 antihuman Eselectin

Antibodies and other agents for in vivo leucocyte labelling:

     Technetium-99m Fab' anti NCA90 [Activated Granulocytes]
     Technetium-99m anti NCA95/CEA [BW250/183]. [Granulocyte
label]
     Technetium-99m anti CD15[S SEA1] [Neutrophil label]
     Iodine-131/123 Styryl Dye [Neutrophil and radiosensitive
lymphocytes]
     Technetium-99m P483H.

Reagents for in vitro leucocyte labelling:

     Indium-111 oxinate
     Technetium-99m HMPAO
     Technetium-99m Colloid

Miscellaneous:
     Fluorine-18 CP99-219 [Fluoroquinolone antibiotic]
```

Figure 1. *Classification of Radiopharmaceuticals utilised to detect foci of infection and inflammation.*

Non-Specific Radiopharmaceuticals.

Gallium-67 Citrate complex.

Gallium[67] Citrate complex has a long history as a radiopharmaceutical. It is commercially available as a ready for use injection, carrier free with a specific activity of around 370MBq/μg. Recommended dose levels for adult patients lie between 74-148 MBq by intravenous injection. Blood clearance is relatively slow and optimal scintigrams are best obtained at 24-60 hours post injection. Gallium accumulates equally well at sites of active infection and in non infected foci of inflammation including sarcoidosis and various pulmonary conditions. It also accumulates in a variety of soft tissue tumours whereby an abnormal focus of Gallium uptake is only indicative of the site of a lesion and not of its nature.

There is evidence that Gallium is present as a negatively charged complex formed with four citrate ions [1]. Its accumulation in soft tissues has been linked to cell membrane permeability [2], DNA levels [3] and, most widely accepted, a transferrin modulated transport analogous to that of iron [4]. The degree of accumulation at sites of infection and inflammation is most likely due to pooling in local oedema combined with binding to phagocytes bacteria and damaged cells in situ.

Indium-111 Chloride.

Indium belongs to the same group of the Periodic Table as Gallium. Indium[111] Chloride is available as a ready for use radiopharmaceutical, carrier free with a high specific activity [1.8GBq/μg] and a pH +/-4. On intravenous injection it binds rapidly to transferrin whilst unbound material oxidises to colloidal form and becomes sequestered in the RES. Indium[111] binding to transferrin is less stable than that of Gallium[67] and its biodistribution is different in having a significant bone marrow component.

Indium[111] Chloride has been used to detect foci of inflammation [5] including osteomyelitis [6]. The administered dose is 74-111 MBq by intravenous injection and scintigraphy is performed at 24-72 hours post injection. In recent years Indium[111] has been more widely used to label leucocytes for the detection of infection.

Cell Labelling.

Leucocytes migrate to sites of infection and inflammation as part of the bodies normal defense response. The concept of using blood cells as a carrier to convey a radiolabel specifically to disease foci is attractive and a number of useful cell labelling techniques have been successfully exploited.

Indium-111 oxine.

Indium[111] for cell labelling is commercially available as Indium oxine [8-hydoroxy quinoline] complex in buffer solution containing tween 80. This lipophylic complex has been widely used to label blood cells including granulocytes, platelets and lymphocytes. Indium labelled leucocytes are widely used for the detection of inflammatory foci [6][7]. The labelling procedure is relatively complicated involving the separation of the cells to be labelled followed by an in vitro labelling and washing procedure. The labelling agent enters the cells by passive diffusion the technical problems lie in the separation and washing procedures. These are discussed in detail elsewhere [8][Sampson this volume]. The recommended dose of labelled leucocytes is 18-37 MBq. The use of Indium oxine has a disadvantage in that the labelling procedure requires suspension of the isolated cells in physiological saline which can affect their viability.

Indium[111] Tropolonate

Indium [2-hydroxy-2.4.6-cycloheptatrienone] as an alternative to the oxine allows the cells to remain suspended in serum which alleviates this problem [9].

Technetium-99m-HMPAO

Technetium-99m-hexamethylpropyleneamineoxine [HMPAO] [Ceretec] a lipophylic complex, developed for imaging cerebral blood flow, readily passes through cell membranes and becomes fixed in the cytoplasm. It is amenable for the in vitro labelling of leucocytes and is probably the most widely used cell labelling agent at this time [10] [11] [12].

Technetium-99m-Colloids

There is a long history of labelling leucocytes with radiocolloids. On incubation with isolated cells or with whole blood the phagocytic neutrophils and monocytes rapidly accumulate and fix the colloid with some detriment to their biological activity. Whilst phagocytosis is a major component of the binding process their is also strong evidence that many of the colloidal particles are retained on the cell surface membrane [13][14]. Whilst simple this method of labelling has not come into widespread use.

Particulate Radiopharmaceuticals.

Technetium-99m Nanocolloid.

Radiolabelled colloids have frequently been observed to accumulate at sites of inflammation. The rapid clearance from the blood pool, of microcolloids designed for liver and spleen imaging, is a disadvantage because the limited exposure time of the lesion to the circulating colloid is too short to permit optimal uptake in the lesion. In addition the particle size of these colloids is relatively large which inhibits extravasation.

In recent years a Technetium-99m albumin colloid with an average particle size of less than 0.1 micrometer and a narrow particle size range has been developed [Nanocoll, Solco\Sorin] which has a slower blood clearance and shows an enhanced uptake at sites of inflammation. This radiopharmaceutical has been extensively used in European centres and has been investigated in detail by De Schrijver [15]

Biodistribution studies in normal rats and in animals with turpentine induced intramuscular abscesses were carried out in the authors laboratory. Electron microscopy of tissue samples, taken at the time of maximum uptake of nanocolloid demonstrated that the colloid readily passed through the damaged capillary membrane and accumulated in the interstitial fluid at the site of the lesion whilst also being scavenged by phagocytes on site. This study also confirmed that nanocolloid particles extravasate through uncompromised capillary walls and enter the interstitial space of normal muscle tissue although to a lesser extent. Similar clinical results have been reported with Technetiun labelled millimicrospheres and this data is also discussed in detail by De Schrijver [15]

Radiolabelled Liposomes.

Liposomes have also been considered as an alternative to labelled leukocytes for the detection of inflammatory foci. It is possible to label them with both Indium-111 and Technetium-99m [16][17]. These are however non specific reagents and the blood clearance is often too rapid to permit adequate exposure of the lesions to allow the liposomes to accumulate. A potential way around this has been the development of so called "stealth liposomes" where the electrical charge on the surface of the liposomes has been neutralised by coating them with polyethylene glycol [18]. This prolongs the residence of the liposomes in the blood stream thereby increasing the exposure time of the lesions to the reagent.

Radiolabelled Antibodies and Peptides.

One of the main drawbacks of using radiolabelled leucocytes for the detection of infection and inflammation is the need to isolate the leucocytes from other blood components to prevent the labelling of other blood cells and plasma proteins. After labelling the leukocytes are washed, to remove unbound radionuclide, before being   re-injected into the patient. The procedure requires special facilities to maintain sterility and stringent protocols to ensure that the patient receives the correct cells when re-injected. The labelling procedure does produce some degree of cell damage and there is evidence that leucocytes labelled in this way are sequestered more rapidly than normal cells.

There has therefore been some interest in developing the possibility of labelling leucocytes in vivo. The development of the technology to produce monoclonal antibodies created the possibility to produce antibodies with a high degree of affinity for cell surface antigens associated with leucocytes. The first images of inflammatory foci with radiolabelled antibodies were reported by Locher [19] who used an Iodine-123 labelled anti-CEA 147 antibody against the human neutrophil antigen NCA95. In a parallel study Joseph [20] reported a similar anti-CEA complex labelled with Technetium-99m which bound to a non specific cross reacting antigen on the granulocyte surface. Further work in this field led to the development of Technetium-99m labelled BW250/183 antigranulocyte complex which has been used extensively in clinical studies [21]. A Technetium labelled anti NCA 90 antigranulocyte antibody [Leukoscan] has been given marketing authorisation in both the

European Union and the USA [22] and is now available for routine use. Technetium-99m labelled anti SSEA1 IGM antibody is also under clinical trial [23].

Non specific uptake of labelled antibodies in the liver, spleen, Kidneys and bone marrow is a problem. to overcome this Rusckowski proposed the application of pretargetting in a similar way to that already used in tumour localisation. Labelled streptavidin localised in E Coli infection foci to the same extent as polyclonal non-specific IgG. Pretargetting with cold streptavidin followed by the injection of Indium-111 labelled Biotin greatly reduced the non-specific uptake in normal tissues and gave an eightfold increase in the lesion to background contrast [24].

An antibody raised against E-Selectin, 1.2B6, has also shown some potential to visualise inflammatory foci [25]. E-Selectin is an endothelial cell specific adhesion molecule for leucocytes and occurs on vascular endotheliun cell surface as part of the inflammatory response. Radioiodinated recombinant Interleukin 1 has been observed to concentrate on receptors at the surface of inflammatory cells and thus in foci of inflammation [26].

Radiolabelled Chemotactic peptides and their analogues have also been proposed as potential imaging agents for focal sites of infection [27]. The labelled peptides retain their receptor binding capacity, their biological behaviour is not significantly altered and importantly it is possible to label with Technetium.

Non Specific IgG

Human non specific polyclonal immunoglobulin labelled with Indium-111 via a DTPA coupling [28], complexed with Technetium-99m N-1-imino-4-mercaptobutyl or Technetium nicotinylhydrazine complex [29][30]. The localisation of nonspecific IgG is primarily due to accumulation in local oedema at the site of inflammation.

Infection or inflammation?

The distinction between inflammation and true infection remains a problem. Rubin [31] investigated the uptake of a radio-iodinated antibody against Fischer immunotype 1 Pseudomonas Aeruginosa and concluded that the direct imaging of Bacterial foci was feasible although he reported non specific uptake at sites of inflammation shortly after injection. Britton [32] took a different approach and has reported encouraging results with a Technetium labelled derivative of the antibiotic ciprofloxacin. The antibiotic is bound specifically by living bacteria where it inactivates DNA gyrase. Dead bacteria and sterile abscesses do not accumulate the complex.

References

1. van der Pompe W.B. An ionic model to explain the distribution of metal chelates in normal and pathological tissues. In: Progress in Radiopharmacology Ed: P.H.Cox. Elsevier North Holland.Amsterdam.[1979] 31-44.
2. Cox. P.H. The biological behaviour of Technetium complexes with particular reference to brain tumours. Ibid. pp 45-62.
3. Taylor D.M. and Hammersley P.A.G. Tumour localisation of Gallium in relation to DNA synthesis, transferrin and lysosomal enzyme activity. Ibid pp 63-73.
4. Hoffer P.B., Bekerman C. and Henkin R.E. Editors. In: Gallium-67 Imaging. John Wiley and Sons, New York.[1978] pp 1-9.
5. Hussein M.A.D. et al. Clinical experience with In-111 Indium Chloride scanning in inflammatory diseases. Clin Nucl Med [1978] 3.196-201.
6. Iles S.E. et al. Indium-111 Chloride scintigraphy in osteomyelitis. J Nucl Med [1987].28.1540-1545.
7. Mountford P.J. et al. A study of leukocyte labelling efficiencies obtained with In-111 oxine. Nucl Med Comm [1985] 6.109-114.
8. Thakur M.L. et al. In-111 labelled cellular blood components; mechanism of labelling and intracellular location in human neutrophils. J Nucl Med [1977] 18. 1020-1024.
9. Peters M.A. et al. Imaging of inflammation with Indium-111 tropolonate labelled leukocytes. J Nucl Med [1983] 24.39-44.
10. Danpure H.J. et al. The development of a clinical protocol for radiolabelling mixed leucocytes with Technetium-99m-hexamethylpropyleneamineoxine [HMPAO]. Nucl Med Comm [1988] 9.465-475.
11. McAfee J.G. et al. 99m-Tc-HMPAO for leucocyte labelling experimental comparison with 111-In oxine in dogs. Eur J Nucl Med [1987] 13.353-357.
12. Roddie M.E. et al. Imaging inflammation with 99m-Tc HMPAO labelled white cells. Nucl Med Comm [1987] 8.285.
13. English D. and Andersen B.R. Labelling of phagocytes from human blood with Technetium-99m sulphur colloid. J Nucl Med [1975] 16.5-10.
14. Mock B.H. and English D. Leukocyte labelling with Technetium-99m Tin colloids. J Nucl Med [1987] 28.1471-1477.
15. De Schrijver M. Scintigraphy of inflammation with nanometer sized colloidal tracers. Kluwer Academic Publishers, Dordrecht.[1989]
16. Beaumier P.L. and Hwang K.J. Efficient method for loading Indium-111 into liposomes using acetylacetone. J Nucl Med [1982] 23.810-815.
17. Goins B. et al. Biodistribution and imaging studies of Technetium-99m labelled liposomes in rats with focal infection. J Nucl Med [1993] 34.2160-2168.
18. Boerman O.C. et al. Tc-99m labelled PEG Liposomes to image infection: Effect of particle size and comparison with Tc-99m labelled leucocytes. Eur J Nucl Med[1996]. 239.1068.

19. Locher J.T. et al. Imaging of inflammatory and infectious lesions after injection of radioiodinated monoclonal anti granulocyte antibodies. Nucl Med Comm [1986] 7.659-670.

20. Joseph K et al. In vivo labelling of granulocytes using Technetium-99m labelled monoclonal antibodies: First clinical results. Nu Comp.[1987] 18.223-229.

21. Becker W. et al. Kinetic data of in vivo labelled granulocytes in humans with murine Technetium-99m labelled monoclonal antibody. Eur J Nucl Med [1989] 15.3611-366.

22. Goldenberg D.M. et al. Use of Leukoscan an antigranulocyte antibody fragment in the evaluation of patients with acute non classic appendicitis. Eur J Nucl Med [1997].24.8

23. Gratz S. et al. 99mTc labelled Anti-SSEA1 murine IGM monoclonal antibodies for imaging infection. Eur J Nucl Med [1996] 239.1067.

24. Rusckowski M. et al. Localisation of infection using streptavidin and biotin; an alternative to non specific polyclonal immunoglobulin. J Nucl Med [1992] 33.1810-1815.

25. Keelan E.T.M. et al. Imaging vascular endothelial activation: An approach using radiolabelled monoclonal antibodies against the endothelial cell adhesion molecule E-Selectin. J Nucl Med [1994] 35.276-281.

26. van der Laken C.J. et al. Specific targetting of infectious foci with radioiodinated human recombinant Interleukin1 in an experimental model. Eur J Nucl Med [1995] 22.1249-1255.

27. Babich J.W. et al. Technetium-99m labelled hydrazino nicotinamide derivatized chemotactic peptide analogues forimaging focalsites of bacterial infection. J Nucl Med [1993] 34.1964-1974.

28. Rubin R.H. et al. In-111 labelled non specific immunoglobulin scanning in the detection of focal infection. N Engl J Med [1989] 231.935-940.

29. Technescan HIG Summary of Product Characteristics. Mallinckrodt Medical. DRN 4369 [1990].

30. Dams E.T.M. et al. Technetium-99m labelled to human immunoglobulin G via the nicotinyl hydrazine derivative [hynic]: first clinical results. Eur J Nucl Med [1996] 239.1068.

31. Rubin R.H. et al. Specific and non specific imaging of localised Fischer Immunotype 1 Pseudomonas Aeruginosa infection with radiolabelled monoclonal antibody. J Nucl Med [1988] 29.651-656.

32. Vinjamuri S. et al. Comparison of Tc-99m Infecton imaging with radiolabelled white cell imaging in the evaluation of bacterial infection. Lancet [1996].347.233-235.

CHAPTER 3

LABELLED CELLS FOR IMAGING INFECTION

Charles B. Sampson

Introduction

The clinical use of radiolabelled leucocytes has been one of the great success stories of nuclear medicine during the past fifteen years. Early work in the USA by Thakur [1] showed that indium-111 oxine could be successfully tagged to white cells and that the technique could be used to determine the sites of infection with high sensitivity and specificity. Later work in the UK [2] confirmed that technetium could also be used as a white cell label provided that is was used in conjunction with the lipophilic chelate hexamethyl propylene amine oxime (HMPAO). Since those early years labelled leucocytes have largely replaced gallium-67 citrate as the method of choice for location of infection and inflammation and the techniques have become widely used throughout the nuclear medicine community.

The labelling of white cells in-vitro has many advantages over labelling in-vivo. For example, the integrity of the label can be checked before injection by removing radioactivity not associated with the cells. Also, the cells can be tested for viability and chemotactic response to ensure that damage has not occurred during the actual labelling process. The most important advantage, however, is that the radioactivity is attached specifically to a biological molecule associated with infection and there is therefore less likelihood of the tracer being taken up at other sites in the body.

This chapter will discuss the essential practicalities of leucocyte labelling and will also consider some of the problems likely to arise during the labelling process it self and after re-injection of the labelled cells. Appendices at the end of the review will summarise the steps needed to label 'mixed' leucocytes with indium and technetium.

P. H.Cox and J. R. Buscombe (eds.), The Imaging of Infection and Inflammation, 31–60.

Chelating agents used in leucocyte labelling.

An ideal leucocyte labelling agent must fulfil several conditions in order to be of use in nuclear medical techniques. Firstly the labelled cells must behave in a similar way to unlabelled cells as it is the chemotactic properties of the labelled cells which are being used to target the radioactivity to specific sites. It is therefore essential that the leucocytes are not damaged during the labelling process. Secondly, the radionuclide used to label the cells must have a half-life which is long enough to allow the clinical study to be completed but not so long that the patient receives a higher radiation dose than is necessary. And finally, the chelate should be of such lipophilicity that it completely crosses the phospholipid bilayer of the cell membrane and remains associated with the cell components during the period of the study. This last factor is of great significance as any radioactivity released from the cells is likely to hamper interpretation of the scintigram by localising in organs or tissues which are not the subject of the investigation. Unnecessary irradiation of these areas will also occur.

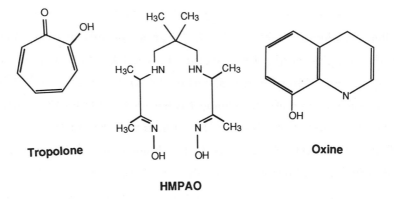

Figure 1. *Some highly lipophilic materials in leucocyte labelling.*

The general approach to successful chelation of leucocytes has been by means of highly lipophilic materials such as those shown in Figure 1.

All of these substances pass into the cell by means of passive diffusion. The first chelator to be introduced for leucocyte labelling was indium-111 oxine which was first used in 1976 [3]. A disadvantage of oxine was that it tended to label the plasma protein transferrin as well as the actual leucocytes. The cell suspension required vigorous washing to remove the plasma and there was a real possibility of cell damage. A more effective cell chelator tropolone, was introduced in 1982 [4] the main advantage being that tropolone does not label proteins. It is also one hundredfold more lipophilic than oxine and is now regarded as the 'gold' standard of indium chelators.

During the 1980's many researchers turned their attention to lipophilic materials that would chelate with technetium and hexamethyl propylene amine oxine (HMPAO [Ceretec, Amersham plc]) became the first commercially available technetium white cell chelator. Whilst its initial intended use was for imaging cerebral blood flow [5] its most widespread use appears to be for leucocyte labelling [6]. The ability of this agent to perform both functions is thought to be due to its instability. The HMPAO complex is neutral and highly lipophilic (log P is approximately 1, [7]). It is thought to be able to cross cell membranes, the react with intracellular components to produce a hydrophilic complex which cannot back diffuse across membranes [5]. In this way technetium is trapped within the cell. It has been proposed that intracellular glutathione is the primary reagent to affect this conversion [8] but after a number of studies there is no firm consensus for or against this hypothesis [9]. Whilst rapid degradation of the complex in-vivo might be essential for efficacy it is a nuisance in the kit. Because of its instability the manufacturer places many restrictions on the use of the kit [10]. For example, the kit must be used for only one patient at a time, the eluate must be freshly prepared and the radioactive concentration must be within defined limits. Many workers have attempted to improve the stability and cost effectiveness of HMPAO and it has been shown that storage in a freezer after reconstitution [11,12] and addition of stannous iron [13] can greatly improve both of those parameters.

Other leucocyte chelators include the heavy metal chelate diethyldithiocarbamate (DDC) which has been successfully chelated with technetium [14] and has been used to label infiltrated leucocytes in cardiac patients [15]. It is surprising that technetium-DDC has not become more widely used as the cost of the chelate is negligible. Of academic interest at present are the hydroxypyranones which have been successfully chelated with indium-111 chloride [16] and which have been used to tag white cells. Hydroxypyranones could, in theory, replace tropolone as a white cell ligand provided that they could be shown to be less toxic to cells than tropolone [17].

Parameters required for successful labelling

Before defining the parameters needed for successful labelling it may be helpful to define what is meant by 'labelling efficiency'(LE) as this is the term used to quantitate the amount of radioactivity incorporated into the cells. To measure the LE the labelled cells should be separated by centrifugation from the medium in which they are labelled. The amount of radioactivity on the cells and the medium is measured and the percentage taken up by the cells is the labelling efficiency. In general the aim should be to incorporate as much of the added radioactivity as possible in order to achieve a high LE provided in doing so the viability of the cells is not compromised. It is important to incorporate that activity at the first attempt as any subsequent re-labelling could damage the cells. It is essential therefore that a labelling method is selected such that the LE is high and that the amount of activity incorporated into the cells is sufficient to produce a good scintigram.

The parameters which affect the amount of radionuclide taken up by the leucocytes are many and varied and are shown in Table 1.

1. The concentration of chelating agent and amount of radioactivity added
2. The concentration of plasma in the labelling medium
3. The cell concentration, cell number and volume of the cell suspension
4. The type of cells being labelled
5. The incubation time and temperature
6. The pH of the labelling medium
7. The presence of drugs in the patient's plasma

Table 1. *Parameters which effect the amount of radionuclides taken up by leucocytes.*

As regards the concentration of chelator and radionuclide, for indium labelling normally up to 18.5 MBq of indium-111 are added to 50 μg tropolone (0.4 x 10^{-6} moles). But 18.5 MBq of indium-111 contains only 10 x 10-12^{-12} moles of indium. Therefore when this metal reacts with the ligand only picomole amounts of radioactive complex are formed [18]. Therefore almost all of the millionfold excess of tropolone does not complex with the radiometal. Some of this non-complexes ligand will react with contaminating stable metal impurities in the radioactive solution. However, most will remain uncomplexed. The concentration of the free ligand affects the amount of radionuclide which is incorporated into the cells possibly by ensuring that the indium remains complexed to the ligand rather than dissociating.

As far as technetium is concerned it was originally thought that 500 μg HMPAO (1.8 x 10^{-16} mols) were needed to form a complex with 450 MBq technetium-99m [18]. However later work [11] showed that the primary lipophilic complex could be obtained by using a much smaller amount of HMPAO. The amount of HMPAO needed for cell labelling could be even further reduced if an additional quantity of stannous ion was incorporated [13].

Turning now to the effects of plasma concentration it has been mentioned previously that if indium oxine is used to label cells in the presence of plasma the label will attach itself preferentially to the plasma protein transferrin. For example, if 10^{-8} granulocytes are labelled with indium tropolonate in 1 ml of 90% plasma a labelling efficiency of 90% is obtained. However, if the same number of cells is labelled in 10 ml plasma at the same concentration the LE decreases to 30%. On the other hand if all the plasma is removed the viability of the cells may be compromised [17], It has been shown that the labelling medium requires only 10% plasma to have a protective effect on cell viability [17]. In practice those who use indium oxine for radiolabelling usually keep the cell suspension in approximately 0.25 ml plasma.

Cell number, cell concentration and volume of ingredients are probably the most important factors which influence LE. The higher the cell number and the cell concentration the higher the LE. In patients known to be neutropenic or leucopenic it is usually a good idea to take a larger volume of blood for labelling. The volume of ingredient will, of course, affect the cell concentration so in practice the volume of the cell suspension and the volume of radioactive fluid must be kept as low as possible. This has been dramatically shown in the case of technetium HMPAO labelled leucocytes [11] when it was demonstrated that if the volume of technetium is kept to 0.5 ml a marked increase in LE is observed.

All the currently used technetium and indium chelators (other than monoclonal antibodies) are non-selective and will therefore label all cell types. For that reason it is essential to remove as far as possible all contaminating cells such as red cells and platelets. It should also be emphasised that in a batch of 'mixed' leucocytes the cell suspension may not be predominantly neutrophils but could be mainly lymphocytes [19] especially if the patient suffers from a chronic inflammatory illness. Because of this phenomenon there has been some discussion within nuclear medicine circles as to whether it might be more clinically accurate to use pure neutrophils and/or lymphocytes for clinical studies rather than mixed leucocytes. The argument for the use of a pure population of cells rather than a 'mixed bag' is further enhanced by the fact that neutrophils and lymphocytes migrate to different locations in some histopathological conditions. For example, in acute bacterial infections there is likely to be a preponderance of neutrophils whereas in diseases of lymphocyte proliferation there will be, of course, be a preponderance of lymphocytes. In many chronic conditions such as inflammatory bowel disease or chronic ulcer there is likely to be large amounts of both cell types. Further complications arise due to the recent discovery of different sub-sets of neutrophils which may have different biodistribution patterns (verbal communication, Dr. J.H. Mehrishi, Cambridge).

As regards temperature as a factor in labelling, cells are usually labelled at room temperature. Cells can be labelled at 37C but there is no evidence that a better label will result if the procedure is carried out at that temperature. If labelled blood is to be stored for one - two hours before re-injection it might be appropriate to store the cells in an oven or portable incubator at 37C. The pH of the labelling is critical and cells should be labelled at pH 7.4 to maintain viability. If acid-citrate-dextrose is used as anti-coagulant the pH of the plasma is lowered to 7.2 but this slight lowering does not seem to interfere with the labelling process or the viability of the cells [18].

Removal of white cells from whole blood

Removal of 'mixed' leucocytes
The first stage in the removal of leucocytes from whole blood is removal of the contaminating red cells by means of a sedimenting agent. Traditional sedimenting agents have included dextran, methylcellulose and dihydroxyethylstarch (hetastarch, Plasmasteril, Hespan). These carbohydrates act by affecting the electronegative of the sialic acid groups on the outer membrane of the red cell. It is thought that some of the cells become more electronegative than their near partners, and they therefore aggregate together to form rouleaux which then sink to the bottom of the tube [20]. Sedimentation is always incomplete as red cells without partners tend to remain floating in the supernatant. It is these red cells which will also take up the label and, if excessive, will show up as blood pool activity on a scintigram.

50 ml of whole blood is taken from the anticubital fossa and immediately anti-coagulated with 6 ml of acid-citrate-dextrose (Formula A, NIH). The syringe of blood should be gently revolved for a few seconds to ensure complete anti-coagulation. The blood is mixed with 10 ml hetastarch or similar sedimenting agent and allowed to stand for up to 60 minutes. Alternatively the sedimentation process can be speeded up by distributing 25 ml blood into each of two tubes containing 5 ml sedimenting agent. The tubes are spun at 14g for 15 minutes. At the end of the sedimentation period the supernatant (platelet-rich, leucocyte-rich plasma) is removed into a 20ml Sterilin tube and spun at 110g for 7 minutes. The supernatant is removed (platelet-rich plasma) and spun at 1000g. The supernatant here is cell-free plasma and is used for dilution of the final injection of labelled cells. The cells at the bottom of the Sterilin tube are predominantly mixed leucocytes and are transferred to a 15ml Falcon tube care being taken not to dislodge the red cells remaining at the bottom of the Sterilin tube. The leucocytes are now ready to take the label (see later). A diagrammatic representation is

shown in Figure 2 below. It should be noted that many factors affect the sedimentation process itself including the number of blood cells, the volume of blood and the presence or absence of disease. Surprisingly, fat globules in the plasma of patient with, for example, hypercholesterolaemia have no effect on sedimentation [21]. Although clinically successful, sedimentation is an arbitrary and passive process and it is difficult to draw up rigid conditions for a completely successful sedimentation.

Separation of pure neutrophils.

Many workers have been able to remove neutrophils from whole blood but a simple method suitable for nuclear medical techniques has recently been reported based on commercially available materials [19]. First, 7.5 ml of a gradient of density 1.119 g/ml

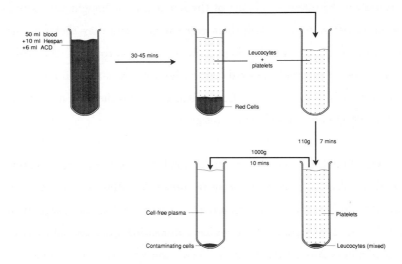

Figure 2. *Steps in the removal of 'mixed' leucocytes from the whole blood*

(Histopaque 1119, Sigma Chemical Co) is poured into a Sterilin Universal tube. 8.5 ml of a gradient of density 1.077 g/ml (Histopaque 1077, Sigma Chemical Co) is then layered carefully over the first gradient. 15ml anti-coagulated whole blood is then poured onto the surface of the gradients care being taken not to disrupt the interface. The tube is spun at 750g for 15 minutes. The second layer, i.e. the neutrophil layer, is removed and washed with cell-free plasma. The purity of the cells has been reported to be in the region of 96%. The procedure will require two or three samples of 15ml blood in order to collect sufficient cells for clinical studies. A diagrammatic representation is shown in Figure 3 below.

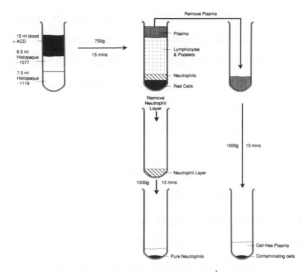

Figure 3. *Steps in the separation of neutrophils from the whole blood.*

Separation of pure lymphocytes.

Lymphocyte scintigraphy could be potentially useful for evaluation of diseases involving chronic inflammation and, possibly, disorders of lymphocyte proliferation. A number of workers have been able to radiolabel lymphocytes with indium but these techniques have not found favour with clinicians because of evidence that chromosomal damage may occur in lymphocytes labelled with that radionuclide [22,23]. A number of workers have proposed technetium as a suitable label and although technetium has been reported to be radiotoxic to lymphocytes [24] cell damage is considerably less than that with indium and it is likely that technetium labelled lymphocytes will become clinically acceptable in the future.

One of the difficulties of using labelled lymphocytes in nuclear medicine is the problem of getting a satisfactory imaging dose of technetium on the small number of cells available. Lymphocytes normally account for only 20-30% of the total number of white cells, 100ml of blood are therefore needed to obtain sufficient cells for clinical imaging. A successful lymphocyte labelling technique was developed in 1991 [25] and the details, briefly, are two 50ml portions of blood are anti-coagulated with acid-citrate-dextrose solution. The blood is transferred to two 50ml Falcon tubes containing Hespan or other sediment agent. The blood is sedimented for 45 minutes and the supernatants collected and spun at 100g for 7 minutes. The supernatants are removed to provide plasma for the final injection. The two plugs of mixed leucocytes are mixed together and made up to 4ml with cell free plasma. The cell suspension is layered onto 3 ml 'Lymphoprep' (Nycomed Laboratories) and spun at 400g for 40 minutes. After centrifugation the first band containing lymphocytes (and monocytes) is removed and washed.

A more recent and simpler technique has been reported in recent years which, again, has been successfully used in clinical studies [26]. 90 mls of anti-coagulated blood are distributed into three 'Accuspin' tubes (Sigma Chemical Co) which have been factory-filled with Histopague of density 1.077 g/ml. The tubes are spun at 100g for 30-40 minutes. The lymphocyte (and monocyte) layer occurs at the top of the tube. The three separate layers are collected together into one tube ready. Any contaminating platelets can be removed by a second centrifugation using a 20% sucrose gradient layered over Histopague 1077. The platelets will remain in the sucrose gradient. The mononuclear cells will be found in the Histopague layer. The mononuclear layer is removed, washed with cell-free plasma and radiolabelled as described below. The advantage of the Accuspin technique is that the prior step to remove mixed leucocytes is not necessary. The Accuspin method is shown diagrammatically in Figure 4.

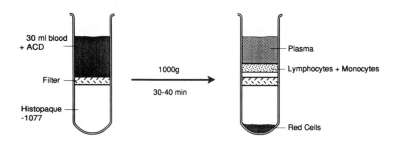

Figure 4. *Steps in the separation of leucocytes from whole blood.*

Radiolabelling procedures

Indium-111 tropolonate

When indium-111 oxine was originally developed many years ago for white cell labelling is was regarded at that time as being the gold standard of cell chelators. With the passage of time, however, and because of the problems alluded to earlier oxine has largely been replaced by tropolone and this section will describe in detail the methodology of labelling with tropolone.

1. Prepare tropolone solution 0.054% according to the following formula:

Tropolone	0.54mg
HEPES	4.77mg
Sodium Chloride BP	8.05 mg
Sodium Hydroxide BP to adjust pH to 7.6	
Water for injection to	1 ml

2. Collect cells to be labelled into a 15ml Falcon tube (cell suspension should be in 0.25ml cell-free plasma).

3. Add 0.1 ml tropolone solution followed immediately by 112-18.5 Mbq indium-111 chloride solution.

4. Incubate for 10 minutes.

5. Remove unbound activity by adding 3ml cell-free plasma and spin at 1000g. Remove the supernatant which is used to determine labelling efficiency.

6. Wash the cells with cell-free plasma.

7. Add 4ml cell-free plasma and suck up the cells into a 10ml disposable syringe. Check the activity. Discard portions of the injection, if necessary, to achieve the required activity. Calculate the labelling efficiency.

8. Transfer the syringe to a lead lined syringe guard and label with the patient's name, hospital number, batch number, date, name of injection and activity at the stated time.

Tc-99m HMPAO

During the past few years many workers have attempted to improve the early work on HMPAO labelling as it had been felt that the original method was time-consuming and not cost effective [27]. Moreover, the original method required as much as 102ml blood from the patient [10]. This could cause problems in patients with poor veins or in children and babies. The following simpler method has been used with great success in thousands of patients and the main steps are shown below.

Add aseptically 6ml sterile nitrogen-flushed saline to a vial of HMPAO('Ceretec', Amersham plc). Store in freezer when not in use (expiry 6-9 months).

2. Add aseptically 6ml sterile saline to a vial of Stannous Medronate (Amersham plc). Take 0.1ml of this solution and make up to 10ml with sterile saline. Stannous solution must be freshly prepared on a daily basis.

3. Prepare the Tc-99m HMPAO solution by taking a 2ml disposable syringe, withdrawing 0.3ml HMPAO solution from above and adding 0.1ml stannous solution to the syringe (via the tip). Add 500 MBq pertechnetate to the contents of the syringe via the tip. To ensure a good label it is essential to keep the volume of pertechnetate small i.e. 0.2 - 0.3ml.

4. Collect the cells to be labelled into a 15ml Falcon tube. Add the Tc-99m HMPAO solution and incubate for 10 minutes.

5. Remove unbound activity by adding 3ml cell-free plasma and spin at 1000g. Remove the supernatant which is used to determine labelling efficiency.

6. Wash the cells with cell-free plasma.

7. Dilute the cells with 4-5mls cell-free plasma and suck up into a syringe to make the final injection. Check the activity. The usual dose for HMPAO white cell imaging is 200 MBq. Discard portions of the injection, if necessary, to achieve the required activity. Calculate the labelling efficiency.

8. Transfer the syringe to a lead-lined guard and label with the patient's name, hospital number, batch number, date, number of injection and activity.

9. Before re-injection identify the patient by at least two parameters.

Selective cell labelling procedures

Major disadvantages of the techniques described above are that they require skilled trained personnel using high-grade laboratory facilities. Also, the operator may be working with infected or potentially infected blood. For those reasons considerable effort has been expended over the years in developing labelling methods where the tracer is selectively taken up by white cells in whole blood without the need for prior removal of the cells.

Colloidal substances such as Tc-99m tin colloid which are phagocytosed by granulocytes but are not incorporated by other blood cells have been used in the past for selective in-vitro labelling of phagocytic cells in whole blood [28]. The original method was based on a commercial kit of tin colloid. The technique was further refined using an 'in-house' method [29] which showed a reasonable degree of clinical success. However, a large number of variables determined the tagging efficiency including the purity of starting materials, the speed at which the colloid was rotated with the blood, and the time the blood was incubated with the colloid. Difficulty in controlling these variables, the reduced viability of the labelled cells was the concomitant release of technetium prevented the method from becoming widely adopted. Also, many workers reported that once the cells has been activated in-vitro they were less effective in the patient as a result of a reduced chemotactic response. But recent success with a commercial kit based on the early 'in-house' formula has recently been reported [30] and a number of clinicians in Europe and the Far East are beginning to adopt the technique. The phagocytotic method, however, has not proved to be quicker to perform than traditional labelling methods as the colloid is required to remain in contact with the blood for up to one and a half hours. A major disadvantage of the method is that the labelled blood will always contain unbound radioactivity which could localise in other organs and hamper the diagnosis.

Selective cell uptake by means of monoclonal antibodies has become an important new field in tracer technology and varied amounts of success have been achieved in recent years. The first to be reported was an anti-granulocyte antibody which has been used with success in Europe [31]. Later developments demonstrated that an indium labelled MOAB could localise onto the CD4 moiety of T-helper lymphocytes. However, the uptake into the lymphocytes was slow and the blood pool activity was high [32]. A more recent development showed that a MOAB against the interleukin-2 receptor on lymphocytes was able to target only those cells which had become activated [33].

Although labelled antibodies have met with success in a few institutions technique has not yet become widely used. It is also costly to perform and the number of centres where antibodies are produced for clinical use is small. Also, there is the risk of an adverse reaction (the 'HAMA' response) with mouse-derived antibodies.

Documentation procedures in leucocyte labelling

The radiolabelling of blood cells is potentially hazardous both to operator and patient. The radiopharmacist is required to be aware of the radiological and the microbiological hazards during processing whilst the nursing and clinical personnel must be aware of the hazards of collecting blood, identifying the patient and re-injecting the radioactive blood. Proper patient identification is a topic which is taken for granted in medical circles and is little written about. However, if errors occur in the administration of blood horrendous sequelae can occur. A recent review noted five instances of error in the nuclear medicine clinic [28]. In one particular incident a patient was infected with a mild form of AIDS as a result of being inadvertently injected with HIV-infected radioactive blood.

Proper documentation is therefore essential to avoid error and the golden rule is to ensure that all tubes which are used in blood manipulation are affixed with at least two unique patient parameters. The system used in the laboratory of the author is shown in Figure 5.

Agranulocytosis	Bone marrow suppression
Asprin	Captopril
Antihistimines	Cholamphenicol
Beta-lacatams	Cytostatics
Captopril	Interlukin-2
Cephalosporins	Penicillins
Chloroquine	Sodium valproate
Co-trimoxazole	
Diclofenac	
Enalapril	*Leukopenia*
Frusemide	
Ibuprofen	Allopurinol
Indomethacin	Beta-lactams
MAO-inhibitors	Carbamazepine
Nifedipine	Cimetidine
Paracetamol	Co-trimoxazole
Penicillins	Gold salts
Rifampicin	Ibuprofen
Tricyclic antidepressants	MAO-inhibitors
Trimethoprim	Mefanamic acid
Vancomycin	Metronidazole
	Penicillins
	Sodium valproate
	Trimethoprim

Table 2. *List of drugs which cause problems with white cell formation and function (adapted with permission from Myler's Side Effects of Drugs)*

A 'Yellow Label' is used which consists of three sections. The first is affixed to the Blood Labelling Day Book and the second portion is affixed to the sedimentation tube.

The third part is fixed to the tray or cabinet where the work is performed. An important feature of the label is its sequential number. At the end of the labelling procedure all three sequential numbers are linked to the patient's name and act as a final check. The Blood Labelling Day Book is a record of all the products used in the labelling procedure and should include the following details.

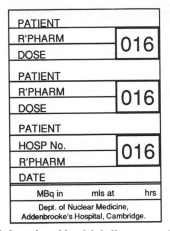

Figure 5. *Three part label used in blood labelling procedures.*

1. Date of procedure

2. First portion of Yellow Label (containing patient's name, radiopharmaceutical and dose).

3. Name of radionuclide, batch number and volume.

4. Name of ligand, batch number and volume.

5. Activity of final injection at specific time.

6. Labelling efficiency.

7. Column for checking the label on the syringe and general documentation.

8. Column for signing by dispenser and checker.

Patient identification at the beginning of the procedure can be carried out by means of two parameters such as name of the patient and birthdate or hospital number. A recent development is the use of bar-coded wrist-straps (Baxter Healthcare Ltd) and this method has been in use in a number of laboratories in the USA. The patient is fitted with a unique bar-coded wrist strap which has a series of detachable duplicate labels.

Each label is affixed to the blood tubes and at the end of the procedure the label on the syringe of radiolabelled cells is tallied with that on the patient's wrist strap. The system is virtually fool-proof for patient identification and could well find flavour in other laboratories.

Problems during radiolabelling

As touched upon earlier the successful radiolabelling of blood cells and their behaviour in the patient is influenced by a large number of factors. These include physico-biochemical factors such as number of cells and cell concentration, methodological factors such as the use of different anti-coagulants and patient-related factors such as drug therapy or the presence or absence of disease. A fuller account of the problems associated with leucocyte labelling has recently been reviewed [34].

Physico-biochemical factors

A good label is dependent on the number of cells present, the cell concentration and the total volume of the cell suspension. If it is suspected that the leucocyte count is low owing to disease it may be appropriate to increase the volume blood taken for labelling to 100 ml. For lymphocyte labelling it is always necessary to use a larger volume of blood. The relevance of cell concentration and volume has been demonstrated by comparing the early method for Tc-99m HMPAO labelling with a recently reported method. In the original technique the amount of ligand required to be added was as high as 4ml [10]. The reported labelling efficiency was in the region of 55%. If however, the volumes of reactants were reduced and the cell concentration increased the labelling efficiency increased to 70-80% [11]. In practical terms it often a good idea to re-elute the technetium generator into a small volume just before the commencement of the labelling procedure to increase the specific activity of the technetium. An added advantage of a method with a high labelling efficiency is that less initial activity is used in the procedure and a consequent reduction in radiation dose to the operator. The sedimentation process is influenced by many physical factors some of which are described by Stokes' Law for a solid travelling through a liquid medium. Although it is outside the scope of this review to discuss the mathematics of sedimentation the process is influenced by the number and density of the particles i.e. red cells, the density of the suspending medium i.e. plasma, the size of the particles and the viscosity of the medium. In addition the number of cells deposited will depend on the volume, circumference and height of the container. For these reasons it is difficult to give hard and fast rules on sedimentation time. The general view is that blood should be allowed to sediment for a maximum of 60 minutes. If left longer there is a possibility that some of the leucocytes will also sink to the bottom of the tube with a consequent reduction in the number available for labelling.

If the red cells do not sediment at all or the time taken for sedimentation appears to be considerably prolonged a number of factors may be responsible. These include incomplete anti- coagulation (see below) or possibly the presence of drugs in the plasma which could affect the red cell membrane. In recent reviews of cell labelling problems versus drugs [35,36] it was observed that out of four reports of difficulties with sedimentation two patients were taking azathioprine and prednisolone, one patient was leukaemic and the fourth patient was being treated with digoxin. Azathioprine disrupts cell membranes as does digoxin so there may be a possible link here. As for the leukaemic patient a second report of a similar occurrence was received soon after the original report so again there may be a causal link. For patient with sickle cell anaemia it is well known that there are difficulties with sedimentation [37].

Cell damage is another factor which can certainly influence behaviour of the cells. If the outer membrane of the leucocyte is disrupted the internal cell proteins will take up the label and are likely to localise in the liver. The correct centrifugation speed is therefore important as is the need to avoid damage during cell washing.

During the collection of lymphocytes the cells sometimes clump together or stick to the inside of the collection tube. The cells should, as far as possible, always be maintained in plasma and if clumps become visible they should be dispersed by slowly drawing through an orange (25G) needle. A number of workers prefer to use siliconised sterile tubes for lymphocyte work to reduce the tendency to stick to surfaces.

Methodological factors

Choice of anti-coagulant can influence cell labelling. Some years ago it was demonstrated that if heparin is used as anticoagulant the labelling efficiency is of the order of 87%. However if acid-citrate-dextrose is used the labelling efficiency increases to 93%.[38]. Anti-coagulation technique in itself can cause problems in the cell labelling laboratory. On a number of occasions it was found in one particular institution that red cells failed to sediment. On close examination of the blood sample small clots were observed. Further investigation revealed that although acid-citrate-dextrose solution was being drawn into the syringe the mixing procedure was insufficient to ensure thorough mixing of all the cells with the anti-coagulant. The general rule is that the syringe should be gently revolved three or four times avoiding frothing of the blood.

Problems sometimes arise during the addition of the radionuclide. It was observed in another laboratory that the labelling efficiency was frequently lower than expected.
On examination of the actual technique it was noticed that the indium was drawn into the pipette 5-10 minutes before it was needed and a very small overpressure in the pipette tip was inadvertently pushing tiny drops of indium out of the tip onto the work tray and so reducing the amount inserted into the cells. Those incidents well demonstrate the need for proper staff training and continuous monitoring of technique.

Patient-related factors

In any busy nuclear medicine department which routinely performs cell labelling procedures unexplainable instances occur where the cells do not adequately take up the label, or the pharmacokinetics of the labelled cells do not correlate either with the presence or absence of disease. A few reports have recently suggested that the patient's own drug therapy may be the cause [35,39]. Although much of the data is anecdotal clinicians and radiopharmacists are beginning to take note of a possible link.

The global pharmacological literature is full of examples of drugs which in themselves produce disease. The number of drugs which affect white cells in particular is extensive; for example, Myler's Side Effects of Drugs lists 42 drugs which cause agranulocytosis, 21 which cause bone marrow suppression and 29 which cause leucopenia [40]. An abbreviated list is shown in Table 2 below.

Evidence that many drugs have a direct effect on the chemotaxis of white cells is irrefutable. For example, the chemotactic response of granulocytes decreased to 60% of its normal value in volunteers taking 40mg prednisone daily [41]. Another study showed that lignocaine inhibited granulocyte adherence by 40% and markedly suppressed the delivery of polymorphonuclear leucocytes to sites of inflammation [42]. Ibuprofen also exhibits similar adverse effects [43] as does vincristine, adriamycin and cyclophosphamide [44]. Both alcohol and aspirin have been reported to affect granulocyte adherence [41].

The question is how important is the drug effect with respect to nuclear medical diagnosis? In an effort to answer this question a survey was recently undertaken in the laboratories of the author to try to assess whether there was a link between patient medication and problems with cell labelling/biodistribution [36]. During an 11-year period 39 adverse reports were received of cell labelling problems. 21 were of unusually low labelling efficiency (<60%) of indium labelled white cells and 9 were of unusually low labelling efficiency (<40%) of Tc-99m HMPAO white cells. On investigation of their respective drug regimes it was revealed that nearly all the patient were being treated with two or more membrane-sensitive drugs such as prednisone, azathioprine, cyclosporin, ranitidine, nifedipine, or metronidazole.

Although much of the clinical data is anecdotal the published in-vitro work on drug-leucocyte interactions together with the clinical findings suggest that there is a real possibility that multi-drug therapy could affect either the labelling process itself or the biokinetics of the leucocytes. The scarcity of data on cell labelling problems emphasises the need for vigorous reporting of adverse incidents and details of the official reporting system are shown at the end of this review.

Quality testing of radiolabelled leucocytes

Many reports have been published of the methods of measuring viability and kinetics of leucocytes such as uptake of the dye Trypan Blue, phagocytosis of bacteria or other particles such as Zymosan and chemotaxis in response to a chemoattractant. Using these methods the effect of radiation, chemical and mechanical damage has been accurately measured [45,46]. However, the important question is how good is in-vitro testing when compared to the actual behaviour of the cells in the patient? An early report compared the random migration and phagocytosis of granulocytes that had been labelled with indium-111 acetylacetone in buffer with indium-111 tropolonate in plasma [47]. Before the cells were injected there was no difference.

However when both sets of cells were re-injected there was a marked difference. The cells which had been labelled in buffer were retained in the lungs for several hours whereas those labelled in plasma were not. The report well illustrates that in-vitro testing may not always correspond with the actual behaviour of the cells in the patient.

Another problem is the time needed to perform in-vitro tests. Cell testing may take as long as 2-3 hours to perform. If the cell procedure takes 2 hours to perform the cells may be out of the body for 5 hours which approaches the 5-6 hour half-life of granulocytes. One would therefore expect to see a deterioration in the cells simply as a result of the time factor.

The most important factor in maintaining high standards in cell labelling is to use properly trained staff and to ensure that rigid written procedures are adhered to. There are, however, several quick and simply quality control measures that can and should be made on labelled leucocytes. The first, the removal of unbound radioactivity, has already been mentioned. Measurement of the labelling efficiency, whilst important, is not always a good indicator of the quality of the "product" as it depends ons o many different factors (see earlier). Thus a low labelling efficiency may be due to either a shortage of cells or drug interference.

Another simple test is to look for clumps or aggregates of cells in the final labelled preparation. This is particularly important with lymphocytes as they have a propensity to clump together. Also, if there appears to be a large amount of red cell contamination in the cell suspension remember that the red cells will also take up the label to produce generalised blood pool activity.

Maltby has recently summarised the most appropriate tests for assessing cell viability [48]. For in-vitro testing the suggests the use of Trypan Blue solution (0.5%) which is taken up by dead cells, promidium iodide which labels dead and dying cells, nitroblue tetrazolium which labels activated cells and the monoclonal antibody CD-45 which tags onto intact cells. He also advocates the use of lung clearance curves (see below) in the first five patients in any new labelling procedure and regular audit consisting of three methods of in-vitro testing together with lung clearance curves.

One of the usual tests to ascertain functional integrity is to observe the biodistribution of the labelled cells during the first 20-30 minutes after injection. Undamaged cells rapidly pass through the lungs and eventually accumulate in inflammatory lesions (and spleen). Damaged cells become trapped in the lungs, show irreversible uptake into the liver and a slow uptake in the inflammatory lesions [47]. Although the test is useful a number of generalised infections also produce margination of leucocytes in the lungs so the results should be treated with caution.

As for the quality testing of lymphocytes most techniques are time-consuming and cannot be used to assess viability before re-injection of the labelled cells. For example, the amount of DNA synthesised after stimulation with a mitogenic agent such as phytohaemagglutanin takes several days to get a result. Other tests such as measurement of chromosome abberations are also useful in assessing the safety of a method at the developmental stage but not for assessing the viability of the labelled cells before re-injection.

Facilities for leucocyte labelling

During the early years when white cell labelling procedures were first performs the general view was that labelling should be carried out within a unidirectional laminar flow cabinet which was sited within an aseptic area. The aseptic area was required to have a standard of air equivalent to Class 2 of BS 5295 (1976). These views were endorsed in the United Kingdom by the Medicines Control Agency [49]. However, with the advent of HIV and the possibility that operators may be working with infected blood new recommendations have recently been made to the effect that cell labelling work should be performed in an isolator [50,51].

Barrier technology by means of isolators is now becoming widespread in radiopharmacy as isolators are specifically designed to project both operator and product. A Type 2 isolator (negative pressure) is specifically recommended for all radiopharmaceutical procedures (including cell labelling) and the isolator is required to be sited within a Class D EC GMP environment [52].

The general use of isolators is outside the scope of this review and further details should be sought in the most recent official publication [53]. However, a few comments might be useful in connection with their use in cell labelling. General sanitization of the cabinet, is of course, essential before commencing the labelling procedure. Sterile 80% IMS is generally regarded as suitable although IMS will not kill blood spores. Other sanitising agents commonly used include sodium hypochlorite solution (keep away from metal surfaces) or Virkon (glutaraldehyde - very potent in killing blood borne bacteria but causes white smears on all work surfaces). All materials should be sprayed with sanitising agent and the labelling procedure should always be carried out on a tray. The tray should be lined with a sterile non-shedding mat.

If the gloving is by means of disposable surgeons' or cytotoxic gloves a glove change is necessary after each radiolabelling procedure. If the gloving is by means of permanent gloves and gauntlets the gloves must be sprayed with sanitising agent after each labelling procedure.

During radiolabelling it is considered bad practice to re-sheath needles after use because of the risk of needle prick injuries. A small "Sharps" container is useful for blood work and should be incinerated at the end of the day as should all non-radioactive blood waste. For disposal of radioactive blood waste technetium labelled waste should be stored in a designated container for three days and then destroyed by incineration. Indium labelled waste should be stored for one week before incineration.

Reporting problems with cell labelling

As discussed previously many of the adverse reports on cell labelling are individual incidents and are somewhat anecdotal. Also, the quantity of published data on in-vivo and in-vitro testing of drugs with pharmaceuticals is currently very small. It is therefore essential to reports and collate all known instances of suspected drug interference. In the European Drug Defect Reporting Scheme cell labelling problems are regarded as a drug defect although, strictly speaking, the defective biodistribution may well be due patient-related factors. An example of the European Drug Defect Report is shown in Table 3 below. Completed forms should be sent to the European collator of drug defects Dr. S. Hesslewood, Regional Radiopharmacy, Department of Medical Physics, Dudley Road Hospital, Birmingham.

APPENDIX I

Indium-111 Tropolonate Radiolabelling of Mixed Leucocytes

1. Collect 50ml blood from patient using a syringe containing 6ml ACD solution (Formula A, NIH).

2. Transfer to a 50ml Falcon tube containing 10ml Hespan (Du Pont) and allow to sediment for 45 minutes. Alternatively split the blood into two 25ml fractions and add each fraction to 5ml Hespan. Spin at 14g for 15 minutes.

3. At the end of the sedimentation or centrifugation process remove the supernatant (WBCs and platelets) and transfer to a 30ml Sterilin tube. Spin at 110g for 7 minutes.

4. Remove the supernatant (platelet-rich plasma)and spin at 1000g. The supernatant (cell-free plasma) is used to dilute the final suspension of labelled leucocytes.

5. The cells at the bottom of the tube from 4 above are mixed leucocytes. Pour these cells into a 15ml Falcon tube taking care to ensure that contaminating red cells remain behind.

6. Spin the leucocytes at 600g to consolidate the plug of cells and remove the supernatant.

UK National and EANM Radiopharmaceutical Reporting scheme

$$\boxed{\text{Confidential}}$$

Details of originator will not be disclosed without express permission. All reports are collated by the EANM Reporting Scheme.

Report of a Radiopharmaceutical Defect

Radiopharmaceutical (Name/code).................................... Manufacturer .... Lot No ....

If relevant:
Radionuclide Generator (Code) .... Manufacturer .... Lot No ....

Date of incident .... Has a commercial manufacturer been informed ? YES/NO

Has MCA been informed (0171 273 0574)? YES/NO

Radiopharmaceutical Defect	Detailed description of the problem:
Tick the appropriate box.	
☐ Transport damage	
☐ Label	
☐ Package insert	
☐ Appearance	
☐ Rad. Surface contamination	
☐ Radioactive Concentration	
☐ Total radioactivity	
☐ Radiochemical purity	Any relevant clinical details of patient(s):
☐ Radionuclide purity	
☐ pH	
☐ Elution Efficiency	
☐ Particulate contamination	Action taken:
☐ Biodistribution	
☐ Sterility/Pyrogens	
☐ Cell labelling	
☐ Other	Supply any further details on a separate sheet.

Report sent by: ....

Address: ....

....

....

Telephone: .... Fax: ....

Send your completed report to:

The Radiopharmacy Assessor,
Radiopharmaceutical Report Scheme,
British Nuclear Medicine Society,
1 Wimpole Street, London, W1M 8AE.
fax 0181 653 9599.

Table 3.

7.   Add 0.1ml tropolone solution followed immediately by the appropriate volume of Indium-111 chloride. The dose of indium for cell labelling is 12-18.5 MBq.

8.   Incubate for 10 minutes.

9.   Remove unbound activity by adding 3ml cell-free plasma from 4 above and spinning at 1000g. Remove the supernatant which is used to determine the labelling efficiency.

10.   Draw up the cells into a 10ml syringe and dilute with 3-4ml cell-free plasma to make the final injection. Check the activity. Discard portions of the injection, if necessary, to achieve the required dose. Calculate the labelling efficiency.

11.   Transfer the syringe to a lead-lined syringe guard and label the guard with Patient's Name, Hospital Number, Name of Injection and Amount of Radioactivity, Time and Batch Number. Affix a "Radioactive" sign to the syringe guard.

12.   Before re-injection identify the patient by at least two parameters.

APPENDIX 2
Tc-99m HMPAO Radiolabelling of Mixed Leucocytes

1.   Prepare stock solutions of HMPAO and Stannous Medronate as described in the text.

2.   Collect 50ml blood from the patient using a syringe containing 6ml ACD solution (Formula A, NIH). Revolve syringe carefully to ensure homogenous anti-coagulation.

3.   Transfer blood to a 50ml Falcon tube containing 10ml Hespan (Du Pont) and allow to sediment for 45 minutes. An alternative method is to split the blood into two 25ml fractions and add each fraction to 5ml Hespan. Spin at 14g for 15 minutes.

4.   At the end of sedimentation or centrifugation remove the supernatant (WBCs and platelets) and transfer to a 30ml Sterilin tube. Spin at 110g for 7 minutes.

5.   Remove the supernatant (platelet-rich plasma) and spin at 1000g. The supernatant (cell-free plasma) is used to dilute the final suspension of labelled leucocytes.

6.   The cells at the bottom of the tube from 5 above are mixed leucocytes. Pour these cells into a 15ml Falcon tube taking care to ensure that contaminating red cells are left behind.

7.   Spin the leucocytes at 600g to consolidate the plug of cells and remove supernatant.

8.   Prepare the Tc-99m HMPAO by taking a 2ml disposable syringe, withdrawing 0.3ml HMPAO solution and adding 0.1ml stannous medronate solution to the syringe (via the tip) Add 500 MBq pertechnetate to the contents of the syringe. To ensure a high labelling efficiency the volume of pertechnetate must be kept as small as possible. It is also essential to prepare the Tc-99m HMPAO first and not add the individual ingredients to the cell.

9.   Add the Tc-99m HMPAO to the cell plug and incubate for 10 minutes.

10.   Remove abound activity by adding 3ml cell-free plasma and spinning at 1000g. Remove the supernatant which is used to determine the labelling efficiency.

11.   Draw the cells into a 10ml syringe and dilute with 3-4ml cell-free plasma to make the final injection. Check the activity. The normal dose for leucocyte scintigraphy is 200 MBq. Discard portions of the injection, is necessary to achieved the required dose. Calculate labelling efficiency.

12.   Transfer the syringe to a lead-lined syringe guard and label with Patient's Name, Hospital Number, Batch Number, Name of Injection and Amount of Radioactivity, Time. A "Radioactive" label should be affixed to the syringe guard.

13.   Before re-injection identify the patient by at least two parameters.

References

1. Thakur ML. Indium-111 labelled leucocytes for the localisation of abcesses: preparation, analysis, tissuedistribution and comparison with gallium-67 citrate in dogs. Lab Clin Med 1977;89: 217-228.

2. Roddie ME. Imaging inflammation with Tc-99m hexamethyl propylene amine oxime (HMPAO) labelled leucocytes. Radiol 1988;166: 767-772.

3. Segal AW, Arnot RN, Thakur ML, and Lavender JP. Indium-111 labelled granulocytes for the diagnosis of abcesses. Lancet 1976;ii: 1056-1061.

4. Danpure HJ, Osman S and Brady F. The labelling of blood cells in plasma with Indium-111 tropolonate. Br J Radiol 1982;55: 247-249.

5. Nowotnik DP, Canning LR, Cummings SA, et al. Development of a Tc-99m labelled radiopharmaceutical for cerebral blood flow imaging. Nucl Med Comm 1985;6: 499-506.

6. Srivastava SC and Straub RF. Blood cell labelling with Tc-99m: Progress and Prospectives. Semin Nucl Med 1990;20: 41-51.

7. Neirinckx RD, Canning LR, Piper IM et al. Technetium-99m d,1-HMPAO: A new radiopharmaceutical for SPECT imaging of regional cerebral blood perfusion. J Nucl Med 1987;28: 191-207.

8. Neirinckx RD, Burke JF, Harrison RC et al. The retention mechanism of technetium-99m labelled HMPAO: intracellular reaction with glutathione. J Cerebr Blood Flow Metabol 1988;8: S4-S12.

9. Babich JW. Technetium-99m HMPAO retention and the role of glutathione- the debate continues. J Nucl Med 1991;32: 1681-1683.

10. Ceretec Package Insert. 1985 Amersham plc.

11. Sampson CB and Solanki. Tc-99m labelled exametazime leucocytes: a high-efficiency multi-dose radiolabelling method using a high concentration and low volume of ligand. Nucl Med Comm;12: 719-723.

12. Sampson CB. Stabilisation of Tc-99m exametazime using ethanol and storage at a low temperature. Proceedings of European Association of Nuclear Medicine Congress, Vienna 1991. Abstract No FP-212-4.

13. Solanki C and Sampson CB. Stabilisation of exametazime for leucocyte labelling: a new approach using tin enhancement. Nucl Med Comm1993;14: 1035-1040.

14. Sampson CB and Solanki C. Technetium labelled leucocytes using diethyldithio-carbamate. Preliminary report on in-vitro studies. Nucl Med Comm 1988; 123-127.

15. McLaughlin AM, Martin W, Tweddel et al. White cells and platelet deposition during cardiopulmonary bypass. Nucl Med Comm 1991;12: 307-308.

16. Ellis B. The development of Novel Bidentate Chelators for Radiolabelling of Cells. Doctoral Thesis 1993. King's College, University of London.

17. Danpure HJ. Cell Labelling with In-111 complexes. In: Theobald AE, editor. Radiopharmacy and Radiopharmaceuticals. Taylor and Francis, London and Philadelphia 1985. 51-85.

18. Danpure HJ and Osman S. Radiolabelling of blood cells-theory. In: Sampson CB editor. Textbook of Radiopharmacy. Gordon and Breach Science Publishers, USA Switzerland 1994 69-74.

19. Sampson CB and Solanki C. Separation and technetium labelling of pure neutrophils: development of a simple and rapid protocol. Nucl Med Comm 1992;13: 210.

20. Sewchand LS and Canham PB. Modes of rouleaux formation of human red blood cells in polyvinylpyrrolidone and dextran solutions. Can J Physiol Pharmacol 1979;57: 1213-1223.

21. Sampson CB and Solanki C. Does plasma fat, viscosity or erythrocyte sedimentation rate affect the radiolabelling of leucocytes? Nucl Med Comm 1989;10: 224.

22. Berge ten RJM, Natarajan AT, Hardeman MR et al. Labelling with Indium-111 has Detrimental Effects on Human Lymphocytes: Concise Communication. J Nucl Med 1983;24: 615-620.

23. Segal AW, Deteix P, Garcia R. Indium-111 labelling of leucocytes: a detrimental effect on neutrophil and lymphocyte function and an improved method of cell labelling. J Nucl Med 1978;19:

1238-1244.

24. Mertz T. Technetium-99m labelled lymphocytes: a radiotoxicity study. J Nucl Med 1986;27: 105-110.

25. Sampson CB and Goffin E. Technetium-labelled autologous lymphocytes: clinical protocol for radiolabelling using a high concentration and low volume of Tc-99m exametazime. Nucl Med Comm 1991;12: 875-878.

26. Sampson CB. Technetium labelled lymphocytes: a plain man's guide to separation and radiolabelling. Nucl Med Comm 1992;13: 400.

27. Sampson CB. Technetium Labelling of Ceretec. Nucl Med Commun 1992;13: 121-122.

28. Schroth HJ, Oberhausen E, Berberich R. Cell labelling with colloidal substances in whole blood. Eur J Nucl Med 1986;6: 469-479.

29. Hanna RW, Lomas FE. Identification of factors affecting technetium-99m leucocyte labelling by phagocytic engulfment and development of an optimal technique. Eur J Nucl Med 1986;12: 159-169.

30. Puncher MRB, Blower PJ. Labelling of leucocytes with colloidal technetium-99m SnF12: an investigation of the labelling process by autoradiography. Eur J Nucl Med 1995;22: 101-107.

31. Locher JTH, Seybold K, Anders REY et al. Imaging of inflammatory and infectious lesions after injection of radiolabelled monoclonal-granulocyte antibodies. Nucl Med Comm 1986;7: 659-665.

32. Becker W, Emmerich F, Horneff G et al. Imaging rheumatoid arthritis specifically with technetium-99m CD4-specific (T-helper lymphocytes) antibodies. Eur J Nucl Med;17: 156-159.

33. Signore A, Parman A, Pozzilli P et al. Detection of activated lymphocytes in endocrine pancreas of BB/W rats by injection of I-123 iodine labelled interleukine-2: an early sign of Type 1 diabetes. Lancet 1987;ii: 536-540.

34. Pharmaceutical and clinical problems with radiolabelled blood cells: a review. Nucl Med Commun 1996 (in press).

35. Sampson CB. Interference of patient medication in the radiolabelling of blood cells: in-vitro and in-vivo effects. In: Sinzinger H, editor. Radioactive Isotopes in Clinical Medicine and Research. 1995 Birkhause, Basel 315-322.

36. Sampson CB. Effect of patient medication on white cell labelling. Br J Radiol 1996 in press.

37. Bunting H. Sedimentation rates of sickled and non-sickled cells from patients with sickle cell anaemia. Am J Med Sci 1940; 191-193.

38. Porter Wc, Dees SM, Freitag JE et al. Effect of heparin and acid-citrate-dextrose on labelling efficiency of Tc-99m labelled RBCs. J Nucl Med 1983;24: 383-385.

39. Sampson CB. Adverse effects and drug interactions with radiopharmaceuticals. Drug Safety 1993;8: 280-294.

40. Myler's. Side Effects of Drugs Annual 17. Editors Aronson JK, Boxted van CJ, 1993. Elsevier, Amsterdam, New York.

41. MacGregor RR, Spaguolo PJ, Lentner AL. Inhibition of Granulocyte adherence by Ethanol, Prednisone and Aspirin measured with an assay System. N Engl J Med 1974: 642-645.

42. MacGregor RR, Thorner RE, Wright DNM. Lidocaine Inhibits Granulocyte Adherence and prevents Granulocyte Delivery to Inflammatory Sites. Blood 1980;2: 203-207.

43. Nielsen VG and Webster RO. Inhibition of polymorphonuclear leucocyte functions by ibuprofen. Immunopharmacology 1987;13: 61-71.

44. Cairo MS, Mallett C, VandeVen C, et al. Impaired In-Vitro Polymorphonuclear Function Secondary to the Chemotherapeutic Effects of Vincristine, Adriamycin, Cyclophosphamide, and Actinomycin D. J Clin Oncol 1986;4: 798-804.

45. Mortelmans L, Verbruggen A, Bogaerts M et al. Evaluation of granulocyte labelling with In-111 chelated to three different agents by functional tests and electron microscopy. J Nucl Med 1986;25: 125-135.

46. Babior BM, Cohen HJ. Measurement of neutrophil function: phagocytosis, degranulation, the respiratory bust and basterial killing. In: Methods in Haematology editor Cline MJ, Churchill Livingstone, London, 1981: 1-38.

47. Saverymuttu SH, Peters AM, Danpure HJ et al. Lung transit of labelled ranulocytes, relationship to labelling techniques. Scand J Haematol 1983;30: 151-156.
48. Maltby P. Methods for assessing white cell viability. Br J Radiol 1966 (in press).
49. Guidance Notes for Hospitals. Premises and Environment for the Preparation of Radiopharmaceuticals in Hospitals. 1982. DHSS London.
50. Institute of Physical Sciences in Medicine. In: Hospital Radiopharmacy Principles and Practice. Frier M, Hesslewood SR, Lawrence R editors. Report No 56 1988.
51. Lazarus C. Design of Hospital Radiopharmacy Laboratories. In Textbook of Radiopharmacy, Theory and Practice. Editor Sampson CB. Harwood Academic Publishers, London, Switzerland 1994: 51-58.
52. The Rules Governing Medicinal Products in the European Cummunity, Volume IV. In: Guide to Good Manufacturing Practice for Medicinal Products, 1989. Brussels, Luxembourg.
53. Isolators for Pharmaceutical Applications. Editors Lee GM and Midcalf B. 1995. HMSO, London.

CHAPTER 4

MICRODOSIMETRY IN LABELLED LEUCOCYTES

Philip J. Blower

Introduction

Several radiopharmaceuticals are now available for the radiolabelling of leucocytes, each with its own putative labelling mechanism and its own technical advantages and disadvantages related to ease of preparation, patient dosimetry, image quality and timing etc. As well as these practical considerations, there are issues of efficacy and safety to consider. There may be immediate effects of the intracellular radioactivity on viability and function (resulting from either the radioactivity itself or from the chemical and physical processing that labelling entails), and there may be long term effects on lymphocytes, which are both potentially proliferative and radiosensitive, leading to risks of leukaemias or lymphomas.

The gamma-emitting radionuclides used to label white cells cause emission of a shower of high-LET Auger and other electrons along with the gamma photon (Table 1 [1,2]). This Auger shower imparts a high radiation dose over a very short range (<1 μm) which is potentially cytotoxic, particularly if emitted from within the cell nucleus [3]. Because of the short range of the high-LET emissions, and because some cellular structures are more radiosensitive than others (the cell nucleus is believed to be the most radiosensitive organelle [3]), the damage from internal radionuclides will depend on their radionuclide properties, their sub-cellular location [1,3,4] and cellular dimensions[5]. Microdosimetry as discussed in this article is the quantification of radiation dose to sub-cellular structures.

The biological consequences of radiolabelling can be measured directly (e.g. by assaying for viability and genetic damage), and the measured effects can, in principle, be correlated with the microdosimetry. The science of microdosimetry is still young, and simple model systems are of value in correlating measurable effects of radioactivity on cells with microdosimetry estimates. That radiolabelled leucocytes (particularly lymphocytes) provide such a model imparts additional value to the study of microdosimetry in leucocytes. For example, the methods used in this simple model can be developed and applied to targeted

61

P. H.Cox and J. R. Buscombe (eds.), The Imaging of Infection and Inflammation, 61–80.
© 1998 Kluwer Academic Publishers. Printed in the Netherlands.

radionuclide therapy for cancer [3,6,7].

Tc-99m			In-111		
E_i (KeV)	n_i	r_i (μm)	E_i (KeV)	n_i	r_i (μm)
0.0334	1.98	0.001-0.01	0.008	7.82	<0.001
0.043	0.019	0.001-0.01	0.039	2.54	0.001-0.01
0.116	0.747	0.001-0.01	0.125	0.915	0.001-0.01
0.226	1.10	0.01-0.1	0.183	0.151	0.001-0.01
1.82	0.991	0.1-1	0.350	2.09	0.01-0.1
2.05	0.087	0.1-1	2.59	0.835	0.1-1
2.32	0.014	0.1-1	3.06	0.190	0.1-1
2.66	0.001	0.1-1	3.53	0.011	0.1-1
15.3	0.013	1-10	19.1	0.103	1-10
17.8	0.005	1-10	22.3	0.039	1-10
119	0.084	>100	25.5	0.004	10-100
122	0.006	>100	145	0.082	>100
137	0.014	>100	167	0.01	>100
140	0.006	>100	171	0.001	>100
			219	0.052	>100
			241	0.009	>100
			245	0.002	>100

Table 1. *Auger and internal conversion electron emissions from In-111 and Tc-99m, giving energy (E_i), number of electrons emitted per disintegration (n_i), and range in water (r_i), Data taken from ref. 1 and 2.*

Direct measurement of the biological consequences of radiolabelling has been attempted in a few instances (discussed below) using assays for viability, proliferative capacity, chemotacticity, and chromosomal damage. The measurements have been of limited value to date: some have not been carried out with clinically relevant levels of radioactivity [8]; few [9,10] have been correlated with microdosimetry; and some have been carried out with leucocyte-labelling agents (e.g. Tc-99m-pyrophosphate [9]) that are not generally used in the clinic and will have different sub-cellular distribution from those that are.

Estimates of microdosimetry have until recently relied on *assumptions* about the distribution of radioactivity within the labelled cells (e.g. a uniform radioactive concentration throughout the cells, or all concentrated at the centre of the cell, or at the cell surface[11]) and among the various types of leucocytes (e.g. the assumption that all labelled cells take up the same amount of radioactivity [11]). These estimates fail to address both the varying radiosensitivity of cellular organelles, and the possibility of non-uniform distribution of radioactivity within the cell. Recent growing recognition of the importance of microdosimetry has led to the development of systems [1] for the calculation of microdosimetry based on *model* geometric distributions of radionuclides in *model* cell geometries (see below). These models require input of information about *real* distribution of radioactivity within the cell to be of significant value. This microdistribution information has recently become available, through the use of techniques such as microautoradiography [6,7] and secondary ion mass spectrometry imaging [12], for some labelling agents in a form suitable for use with the models.

Microdosimetry of radiolabelled leucocytes is discussed here in relation to three commonly used leucocyte-labelling radiopharmaceuticals: In-111-oxine, Tc-99m-HMPAO (Exametazime), and Tc-99m-labelled stannous fluoride colloid. The microdosimetry discussion focusses principally on *lymphocytes* because of the availability of a suitable model for these cells, and because they alone are both radiosensitive and proliferative [13,14,15].

Microdosimetry of In-111 and Tc-99m: radionuclide properties

In-111 has a greater potential than Tc-99m to inflict radiobiological damage both close to the site of deposition (< 0.1 μm) and remote from it (up to the diameter of the cell) because of its greater yield of extra-nuclear electrons per disintegration, both at very low and high energy (Table 1) and because of its longer half-life (68 h, c.f. 6 h for Tc-99m). This is to some extent mitigated by the lower levels of radioactivity used for radiolabelling with In-111 (e.g. 15 Mbq, c.f. 200 MBq for Tc-99m). These levels of radioactivity are determined principally from traditional macrodosimetry considerations: thus, although image quality is better with Tc-99m, higher activities are used because it is perceived as safe to do so as Tc-99m has a short half-life. In addition to these distinctions, it is necessary to account for the possibility that the radioactivity is distributed within and among the leucocytes differently for each radiotracer. Until now, no attempt has been made to include the latter contribution. Information about this radioactivity distribution ("microdistribution") is

included in this article and used in conjunction with microdosimetry models [1] to give
quantitative microdosimetry estimates.

	In-111	Tc-99m
activity in nucleus	8.6×10^{-7}	4.5×10^{-7}
activity in cytoplasm	1.7×10^{-7}	0.2×10^{-7}
activity in membrane	7.9×10^{-4}	0.8×10^{-4}

Table 2 *Summary of calculated dose rates to the centre of the nucleus of a model lymphocyte
from radioactivity localised at a concentration of 1 MBq₋₃cm uniformly in the nucleus only or
cytoplasm only, 1 MBq cm⁻² on the plasma membrane only [1]*

The model lymphocyte doses are expressed as dose rates to the organelle from radioactivity
uniformly distributed in nucleus, or cytoplasm, at a concentration of 1 MBq cm⁻³, or from
radioactivity uniformly distributed over the cell surface at a density of 1 MBq cm⁻² [1]. The
dose rates can be expressed as a single dose rate at the centre of the nucleus (Table 2) or as
a dose rate profile across the cell, such as that shown in Fig. 1 for In-111 in the cell nucleus.
Similar diagrams have been produced for radioactivity localised in cytoplasm and on the
cell membrane[1].

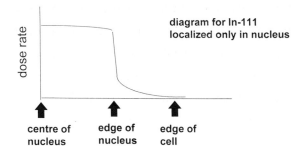

Figure 1. *Schematic representation of the dose rate profile across a model lymphocyte with In-
111 uniformly distributed within the cell nucleus only. Analogous diagrams are available for
other radionuclides and other limiting distributions (uniform distribution in cytoplasm only
and uniform distribution on plasma membrane only) [1]*

Microdistribution of tracer in labelled leucocytes

Indium-111-oxine. Indium oxine is characterised as an uncharged lipophilic complex which enters cells rapidly by diffusion through the lipid bilayer membrane, and subsequently dissociates allowing the indium to bind to intracellular components [16]. The nature of the binding is unknown but is probably related to the "hard" nature of the In^{3+} cation: phosphates, for example, might provide suitable binding sites.

There is no selectivity of the tracers for any particular type of leucocyte [17]. However, there is not a consensus in the literature about the sub-cellular distribution of the In-111 in In-111-oxine-labelled leucocytes: cell fractionation results suggest principally cytoplasmic uptake [16], while principally nuclear uptake is suggested by electron microscope autoradiography [18] and light microscope autoradiography [17]. The cell fractionation results [16] suffer from uncertainty as to whether radionuclide redistribution may have occurred as a result of cell fragmentation, and from the absence of quantitative measurements of radioactivity in cell nuclei. The electron microscope autoradiography [18] was carried out on macrophages and not on circulating leucocytes, and again suffers from uncertainty that the radionuclide distribution observed may not accurately reflect that *in vivo* because of the extensive sample preparation involved in electron microscope autoradiography. The light microscope work [17] was done with sectioned frozen cells, which gives confidence that the radionuclide distribution is realistic, but the histological quality is impaired by freezing. Nevertheless this method has probably provided the most statistically reliable results over the range of cell types present in "mixed leucocyte" samples.

The latter study confirmed that the mean cellular radioactive concentration was the same for all cell types (Table 3). This means, of course, that the larger cells (granulocytes) will contain more radioactivity per cell than the smaller ones (lymphocytes). However, the cellular radioactive concentration in a population of cells was not distributed normally about the mean: about half the cells contained little or no radioactivity, while the other half were very heavily labelled (Fig. 2)[17]. Thus, for In-111-oxine, the *mean* cellular radioactivity should be treated with caution in dosimetry and risk evaluation.

The distribution within cells, as evaluated by light microscope autoradiography, was

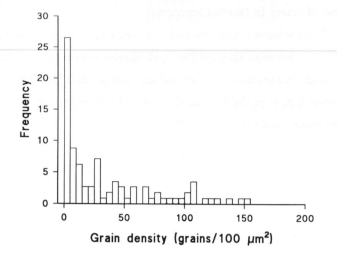

Figure 2. *Distribution of radiolabel among In-111-oxine labelled leucocytes in a sample labelled by a standard clinical protocol. No distinction is made between different types of leucocytes. Cells are categorized into intervals of grain density (which is proportional to radioactivity concentration in the cells). Vertical axis represents the relative numbers of cells in these intervals [17].*

confirmed by isolation of cell nuclei [17]. A ratio of 2.2:1 was found for the nuclear:cytoplasmic radioactivity concentration for all cell types (Table 3). This is the value immediately after labelling, and no determination of the distribution at later times has been done. This ratio can be used, together with data for typical clinical use of In-111-oxine (the typical injected radioactivity, 15 MBq, and leucocyte number, 4 x 10^8, and the typical lymphocyte content of a leucocyte sample, 30%), to estimate the mean absolute concentration in cytoplasm and nuclei. That lymphocytes are smaller than granulocytes (relative volume 0.58 compared to neutrophils [17]) must also be taken into account. These concentrations are required as input into the models provided by Faraggi and co-workers [1] to calculate the microdosimetry. The results are listed in Table 4. At this point, suffice to say that the nuclear selectivity will lead to a higher nuclear radiation dose than that predicted by the assumption of uniform sub-cellular distribution but lower than the unrealistic model of all radioactivity located as a point source at the centre of the cell [11].

	In-111-oxine	Tc-99m-HMPAO	Tc-99m-SnF$_2$ colloid
cell selectivity	none	eosinophils[a]	neutrophils[b]
sub-cellular selectivity	nucleus[c]	uniform	membrane (lymphocytes) cytoplasm (neutrophils)
aggregation	all labelled neutrophils	none	none

Table 3. *Summary of cell type selectivity and sub-cellular distribution of In-111-oxine, Tc-99m-HMPAO, and Tc-99m-SnF$_2$ colloid. a: Fig.3; b: see Fig.6; c: nuclear: cytoplasmic radioactive concentration ratio was 2.2:1 for all cell types.*

Tc-99m-HMPAO. Like In-111-oxine, Tc-99m-HMPAO is a lipophilic species which is believed to enter cells non-selectively by diffusion across membranes. Some form of instability leads to its intracellular binding, but to what is unknown. There is general agreement that Tc-99m-HMPAO shows no selectivity for the cell nucleus. Several techniques provide evidence for this: secondary ion mass spectroscopic imaging of the distribution of elemental technetium [12], cell fractionation studies [19], and microautoradiography [20] all demonstrated uniform sub-cellular distribution of technetium-99m. However, the radioactivity is not evenly distributed among cells: although unlike In-111-oxine, Tc-99mHMPAO was normally distributed among cells of a given type, it was highly selective for eosinophils compared to neutrophils and lymphocytes (Table 3)[20]. The extent of this selectivity is shown in Fig. 3. The radioactivity concentration in neutrophils did not differ significantly from that in lymphocytes. These conclusions were reached on the basis of microautoradiography and density gradient separation of neutrophils, lymphocytes and eosinophils[20]. Except in rare cases, eosinophils comprise only a small fraction of leucocytes (2-4%) in circulating blood. At this level, only about 10-15% of radioactivity in the labelled leucocytes is in eosinophils, and the assumptions of uniform sub-cellular distribution and normal distribution among leucocytes are reasonable. Again, by combining data for typical use of Tc-99m-HMPAO (200 MBq injected dose, 4 x 10^8 leucocytes, 30% of which are lymphocytes) the cytoplasmic and nuclear radioactivity concentrations can be estimated. The estimates are shown in Table 4.

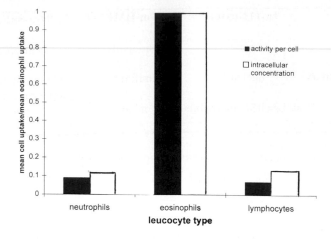

Figure 3. *Selectivity of Tc-99m-HMPAO for eosinophils in a mixed sample. Vertical axis represents ratio of mean uptake in a cell type (neutrophils, eosinophils, lymphocytes) to that in eosinophils. Uptake is measured either as total radioactivity per cell (left column) or as radioactivity concentration in cells (right column). These ratios are different because of the different means volumes of the different cell types [2].*

Tc-stannous fluoride colloid. Tc-99m-stannous fluoride colloid is a particulate radiopharmaceutical that is now commercially available in a form suitable for leucocyte labelling (Radpharm Scientific, Australia). This agent was introduced in order to avoid the need to isolate leucocytes from whole blood prior to labelling. It is claimed that leucocyte selectivity, by phagocytic uptake, is achieved in whole blood [22,23], but this is disputed by other workers who found that most of the activity is bound to erythrocytes [24]. Again, *in vitro* methods on the bulk leucocyte sample suggested that the cells were viable and retained chemotactic activity. Initial studies showed that the leucocyte population as a whole was viable and chemotactic[22], but since only a small fraction of the neutrophils present are labelled[25], this is an insufficiently sensitive assay. The chemotacticity of those cells in the population that have ingested or bound radioactivity must be determined. This was done by Mock and English [24] who showed that the labelled cells were indeed viable and chemotactic. However, no direct quantitative chemotacticity comparison between labelled and unlabelled cells has yet been carried out, so the extent to which radiolabelling affects the cells' behaviour remains uncertain.

This system has also been studied by autoradiography[25], using cells labelled both in whole blood, as indicated by the manufacturer, and in purified leucocytes. Autoradiographs showed two types of labelling pattern: the one shown in Fig. 4 with a concentrated focus of silver grains at the edge of a cell. This pattern is due to a particle at the cell surface. With the cells in focus, it is clear that this is an eosinophil. Lymphocytes too showed exclusively this pattern of labelling. The other type was a more diffuse pattern (Fig. 5), due to radioactivity inside the cell and therefore not in direct contact with the radiographic emulsion.

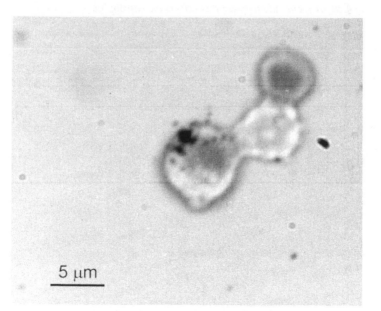

Figure 4. *(a) Microautoradiograph of an eosinophil (in a mixed leucocyte sample) labelled with Tc-99m-SnF₂ colloid. The radioactive colloidal particle is seen adhering to the edge of the cell. A: silver grains in focus, showing focal nature of silver grain cluster due to radioactivity in direct contact with emulsion.*

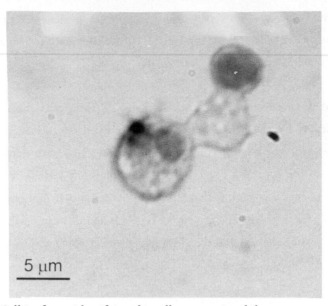

Figure 4. *(b) Cell in focus, identifying this cell as an eosinophil.*

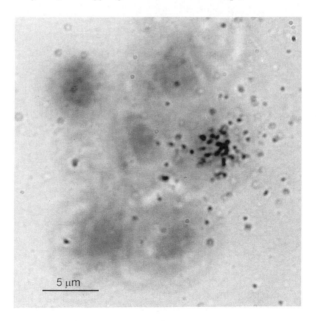

Figure 5. *(a) Microautoradiograph of a neutrophil (in a mixed leucocyte sample) labelled with Tc-99m-SnF₂ colloid. The radioactive particle is inside the cell and gives a focal pattern of silcer grains in the autoradiograph as only the higher ernergy electrons reach the emulsion. A: Silver grains in focus.*

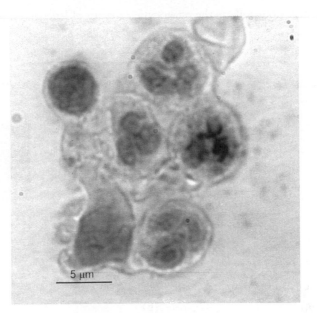

Figure 5. *(b) Cell in focus, identifying cell as a neutrophil.*

The cell selectivity of the colloid is illustrated in pie charts in Fig. 6A-D. Fig. 6A shows the cellular composition of the whole blood (almost all erythrocytes) while Fig. 6C shows that of leucocyte-rich plasma (LRP): a little over 50% erythrocytes. Fig. 6B shows the distribution of radioactivity among the cell types in whole blood: only about 75% of the radioactivity was in erythrocytes. Thus, some selectivity for leucocytes is expressed, but hardly the claimed 80%. In LRP (Fig. 6D) over 90% of the radioactivity was in leucocytes, and about 83% of that was in neutrophils. This is a much greater neutrophil selectivity than when labelling whole blood, and also a greater neutrophil selectivity than achieved with the other radiolabelling agents. The neutrophil selectivity is expressed differently in Fig. 7. The *percent of each cell type that become labelled* is shown: this is a measure of the cells *relative affinity* for the colloid. The neutrophils have a higher relative affinity than the other leucocytes, and very much higher than erythrocytes. Fig. 7 also shows the relation between the relative affinity and sub-cellular location. It charts the percent of each cell type labelled inside the cell or on the surface. Over 90% of the neutrophils and some monocytes (the small number of the latter precluded accurate determination) show the intracellular pattern, while the other leucocytes, and erythrocytes, show only surface

binding. This behaviour reflects the phagocytic capacity of leucocytes: the neutrophils are
the predominant phagocytic cells.

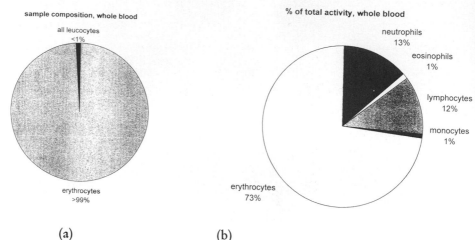

(a)   (b)

Figure 6. *Pie charts showing selectivity of Tc-99m-SnD$_2$ colloid for blood cell types [25].   A:
cellular composition of whole blood sample.   B: distribution of radioactivity among blood cell
types labelled whole blood sample.*

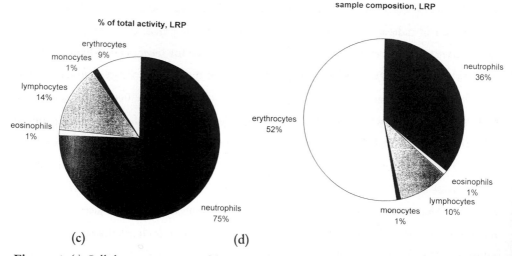

(c)   (d)

Figure 6 *(c) Cellular composition of leucocyte-rich plasma (LRP) sample; (d) distribution of
radioactivity among cell types in a labelled LRP sample.*

Once again, the distribution data can be used in conjunction with data on typical clinical usage. However, because of the very small fraction of lymphocytes that become labelled (4% of lymphocytes in LRP, and much less in whole blood), and the extremely concentrated nature of the radioactivity in the colloidal particles, the mean radioactivity per lymphocyte is a highly inappropriate quantity to use. Instead, the mean radioactivity attached to those few lymphocytes that do become labelled is calculated. This is based on an estimate of the mean radioactivity per colloidal particle (61 Bq, calculated from the experiments with LRP labelling[25] and the observation that no lymphocytes were found with more than one adhering particle[25].

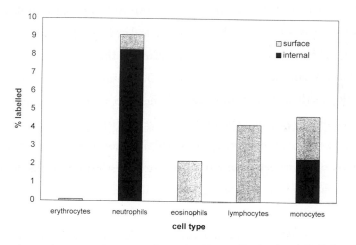

Figure 7. *Pie charts showing selectivity of Tc-99m-SnF₂ colloid when labelled in leucocyte-rich plasma (LRP) [25]. The % of each cell type labelled is taken as a measure of its affinity for the colloid. The total height of each bar represents labelled cells irrespective of subcellular location. The dark shading represents cells labelled internally (phagocytosis). The Grey shading represetns cells labelled "non-specifically" by surface adherance.*

It is obvious that the dose to the nucleus from radioactivity bound to the cell surface is much less than that from the same amount of intracellular radioactivity because the nucleus is beyond the range of most electrons emitted from the cell surface. However, the higher injected radioactivity, the smaller number of labelled lymphocytes, and the extremely high concentration of the surface bound radioactivity may compensate for this: the quantitative results are shown in Table 4. The calculations are based on an injected radioactivity of 500

MBq, in the form of whole blood containing 4.7×10^7 leucocytes, 30% of which are lymphocytes.

Microdosimetry calculations

Having estimated the regional sub-cellular radionuclide concentrations resulting from typical labelling procedures with the three radiotracers, it is now possible to use the estimates to calculate the radiation dose to the cell nucleus, cytoplasm and membrane in labelled cells. This discussion focusses on the nuclei of labelled lymphocytes.

For cells labelled with In-111-oxine and Tc-99m-HMPAO, the radiation dose rate at the centre of the nucleus for real labelled cells is calculated by scaling the dose rate from nucleus and cytoplasm (values in Table 2) according to the true mean concentrations in these compartments, and summing these scaled contributions. For cells labelled with Tc-99m-colloid, this method is inappropriate and the dose at the centre of the nucleus is calculated by assuming that the radioactivity in the adhering particle is uniformly spread over the cell surface, as required by the model. This is reasonable for estimation of the dose rate at the centre of the nucleus, but not, of course, for estimation of the dose rate to the cell membrane, since the latter will be highly non-uniform. The results are shown in Table 4.

The total dose nuclear dose for Tc-99m-HMPAO (0.054 Gy MBq^{-1} for 4×10^8 cells) is in remarkably close agreement to the whole cell dose obtained for Tc-99m-pyrophosphate-labelled lymphocytes (0.19 Gy MBq^{-1} for 10^8 cells)[9]. When corrected for the different cell numbers employed in the calculation, the latter is equivalent to 0.049 Gy MBq^{-1} for 4×10^8 cells. The nuclear dose rate per MBq of injected radioactivity is higher for In-111-oxine than for Tc-99m-HMPAO, partly because of the greater Auger electron yield, and partly because of the selective accumulation in the nucleus. In many In-111-oxine-labelled cells the nuclear dose rate will be much higher still because of the non-normal distribution of radioactivity among cells, while in others it will be much lower. The radiolabel is normally distributed among lymphocytes in Tc-99m-HMPAO-labelled populations, so the number of cells subjected to extremely high or low dose rates is less than for In-111-oxine. The longer half-life of In-111 compounds the difference and the total dose per MBq delivered to the nucleus during the lifetime of the cell is much higher than for Tc-99m-HMPAO. However, because the administered activity of Tc-99m-HMPAO is higher (and therefore, mean activity per cell is higher), the total nuclear dose for In-111 is only about twice that for Tc-99m. The assumption that the radioactivity remains in the cell for infinite time is an approximation that will be more inaccurate for the longer half-life In-111. If this is qualitatively taken into account it appears that the dose to the lymphocyte cell nucleus in clinically appropriate samples of labelled leucocytes is of the same order whether the radiolabel is Tc-99m-HMPAO or In-111-oxine.

For cells labelled with Tc-99m-colloid, which is bound to the surface of lymphocytes, it might be expected that because the radioactivity is located relatively remote from the centre of the nucleus, the dose rate at that point would be very small. However, the particulate nature of the tracer means that the radioactive concentration is extraordinarily high on a labelled cell, but that a very small fraction of cells are labelled. Thus, even the relatively few higher energy electrons per decomposition are sufficient to cause very high radiation dose rates at the nuclear centre. Despite the fact that no Tc-99m is deposited in the nucleus or cytoplasm, the nuclear dose rate is the highest of all the tracers. The dose rate to the cell membrane at the point of adherence is very large indeed, and the radiobiological effects of this cannot be neglected (but equally, cannot be predicted).

Radiobiological effects

These dosimetry consideration have to be placed alongside measurement of the radiobiological consequences of labelling if effects on cellular function and proliferativity, survival, and risk of malignancy are to be optimised and mechanisms of radiation damage are to be understood. The microdosimetry merely provides a means of measuring the radiation doses that give rise to these consequences and are not predictive in themselves. It has been suggested that because of the low likelihood of proliferation of lymphocytes in the body, together with the reduced likelihood of survival after labelling and the small number of injected lymphocytes as a fraction of the total body lymphocyte population, that the risk of malignant transformation is very remote[14].

Some attempts have been made to determine the radiobiological consequences of labelling, both short-term and long-term. Radiolabelling leucocytes with In-111-oxine leaves the

P.J. BLOWER

granulocyte function apparently unimpaired, or only transiently impaired.

	In-111-oxine	Tc-99m-HMPAO	Tc-99m-SnF$_2$ colloid
injected dose, MBq	15	200	500
no. of cells injected	4.0×10^8	4.0×10^8	4.7×10^7
nuclear concentration, MBq cm^{-3}	69	732	0
cytoplasmic concentration, MBq cm^{-3}	31	732	0
cell membrane concentration, MBq cm^{-2}	0	0	19
[a]initial nuclear dose rate, Gy s^{-1} MBq^{-1}	4.0×10^{-6}	1.7×10^{-6}	n.a.[e]
[b]initial nuclear dose rate, Gy s^{-1}	6.0×10^{-5}	3.4×10^{-4}	1.6×10^{-3}
[c]total nuclear dose, Gy MBq^{-1}	1.4	0.05	n.a.[e]
[d]total nuclear dose, Gy	21	11	48

Table 4. *Quantitative estimates of dose rates and doses to nuclei of lymphocytes based on both measured sub-cellular distribution and model dosimetry [1]. Typical injected radioactivity dose and number of cells on which calculation is based are also included. a: dose rate to nucleus immediately after labelling, per MBq of injected radioactivity; b: dose rate to nucleus immediately after labelling typical labelling; c: total integrated dose to nucleus assuming infinite cell biological lifetime, per MBq of injected radioactivity; d: total integrated dose to nucleus assuming infinite cell biological lifetime, after a typical labelling; e: not applicable: this parameter is not valid for Tc-99m-SnF$_2$ colloid because of extremely high radioactivity uptake by extremely few lymphocytes.*

Some effects have been noted: a degree of activation is indicated by increased initial margination in lung[26], and by aggregation of neutrophils[25]. The degree of aggregation is highly correlated with the radioactivity concentration in the cells (Fig. 8), suggesting a radiobiological effect. However, chemical effects could equally be responsible for causing aggregation[25]. The effects on lymphocytes are more severe. Lymphocytes are highly radiosensitive, and levels of In-111-oxine below 5 MBq per 10^8 cells markedly reduced recirculation and localisation in lymph nodes [13].

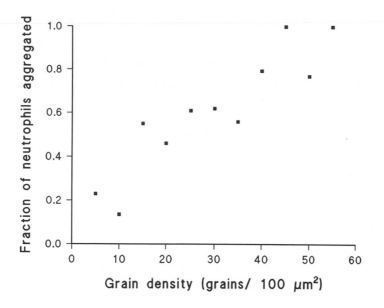

Figure 8. *Correlation of radioactive concentration within leucocytes with the probability that the neutrophil is part of an aggregate. Data are taken from several thousand cells within one sample of labelled neutophils [17].*

Long-term genetic effects are also apparent: chromosomal abnormalities are very frequent among dividing In-111-labelled lymphocytes, even at sub-clinical labelling levels[27]. The mean uptake per cell in a typical clinical labelling procedure is of the order of 0.02-0.1 Bq (range spanned by data from our work and others[28]). Lymphocytes suffer chromosome damage following labelling levels at least an order of magnitude lower than this[27].

Tc-99m-HMPAO-labelled leucocytes of any type do not aggregate after labelling with typical clinical levels of activity[20]. However, once again genetic damage is detectable in lymphocytes labelled with Tc-99m-HMPAO [8] or Tc-99m-pyrophosphate [9]. At a labelling level of about 200 MBq Tc-99m-pyrophosphate per 10^8 cells (roughly equivalent to clinical level) both cell division delay and chromosome damage were observed. At twice this level no lymphocytes survived[9]. Likewise, in lymphocytes labelled with Tc-99m-HMPAO there is substantial chromosome damage even at labelling levels well below the clinical level[8]. At levels about 4 fold higher than the typical clinical imaging level, the lymphocytes no longer proliferate, so malignant transformation is impossible. What happens in between, at the levels of activity normally used, is not reported. If the microdosimetry results have any predictive value, the biological effects should be similar to those of labelling with In-111-oxine at clinically appropriate levels. The chromosome damage inflicted by the intracellular radioactivity at a typical clinical level (200 MBq per 4×10^8 leucocytes) was estimated to be equivalent to about 7 Gy of external X-rays. This is remarkably close to the calculated dose to the nuclei of Tc-99m-HMPAO labelled cells (Table 4), and suggests a degree of equivalence between internal and external radiation doses.

A point of concern is what fraction of genetically damaged cells survive and are proliferative[27,29]. The radiobiological results [8,9] suggest that because of the inhibition of division associated with radiolabelling at clinical levels with Tc-99m-pyrophosphate, the conclusion of Wagstaff [14] is warranted: the probability of proliferation is very low and the risk of malignant transformation is negligible.

These radiobiological studies are very limited and more are required to characterise adequately the effects of labelling on lymphocytes. There have been no radiobiological studies at all on Tc-99m-colloid-labelled lymphocytes. It may be difficult to remedy this, because the label may be insufficiently strongly bound to the cell surface for prolonged tracer experiments: it has been shown that erythrocytes "non-specifically" labelled by surface adhesion of the colloid easily lose their radiolabel to neutrophils within a short time *in vitro*[25].

Conclusions

A summary of the cell selectivity and sub-cellular distribution is shown in Table 3, and estimates of the radiation doses to the nuclei of lymphocytes for each tracer are shown in Table 4. The short term and long term radiobiological consequences of reinjecting labelled leucocytes, whether they affect the efficacy of the imaging technique or the long-term risk of malignancy, are expected to depend on the microdosimetry of the labelled leucocytes. This in turn depends on the nature and amount of radionuclide used, and its distribution among and within cells as a function of time. The time dependence of sub-cellular distribution has not yet been studied to a significant degree. The microdistribution studies have shown that it is inappropriate to assume uniform distribution among and within cells. Each labelling agent has its own sub-cellular distribution and cell selectivity (Table 3). By taking into account sub-cellular distribution and coupling this data with microdosimetric models it is possible to obtain estimates of radiation doses to different organelles, of which the nucleus is believed at present to be the most important. This information can in principle be combined with radiobiological experiments that directly measure the consequences of radiolabelling, in order to improve understanding of the effects of intracellular radioactivity on sub-cellular structures. This is of particular interest for lymphocytes, but the results could help illuminate our current relatively hit-and-miss approaches to targeted radionuclide therapy, and identify and quantify any risks of malignancy arising from incorporation of radioactivity into potentially proliferative cells such as germ cells[4], lymphocytes[14] and nascent blood cells in the bone marrow.

References

1. Faraggi M, Gardin I, de Labriolle-Vaylet C, Moretti J-L, Bok B. The influence of tracer localization on the electron dose rate delivered to the cell nucleus. J Nucl Med 1994;35:113-119.
2. Jonsson B-A, Strand S-E, Emanuelson H, Larsson B. Tissue, cellular and subcellular distribution of indium radionuclides in the rat. In: Howell RW, Narra VR, Sastry KSR, Rao DV, editors. Biophysical Aspects of Auger Processes (AAPM Symposium series). New York: American Institute of Physics; 1992:249-272.
3. Hofer KG, Harris CR, Smith JM. Radiotoxicity of intracellular 67Ga, 125I, and 3H: nuclear versus cytoplasmic radiation in murine L1210 leukaemia. Int J Radiat Biol 1975;28:225-241.
4. Rao DV, Narra VR, Howell RW, Lankha VK, Sastry KSR. Induction of sperm head abnormalities by incorporated radionuclides: dependence on subcellular distribution, type of radiation, dose rate, and presence of radioprotectors. Radiat Res 1991;125:89-97.
5. Gardin I, Faraggi M, Huc E, Bok B. Modelling of the relationship between cell dimensions and mean electron dose delivered to the cell nucleus:application to five radionuclides used in nuclear medicine. Phys Med Biol 1995;40:1001-1004.
6. Humm JL, Machlis RM, Bump K, Cobb LM, Chin LM. Internal dosimetry using data derived from autoradiographs. J Nucl Med 1993;34:1811-1817.
7. Puncher MRB, Blower PJ. Radionuclide targeting and dosimetry at the microscopic level: the role of microautoradiography. Eur J Nucl Med 1994;21:1347-1365.
8. Thierens HMA, Vral AM, van Haelst AM, van de Wiele C, Schelstraete KHG, de Ridder LIF. Lymphocyte labeling with technetium-99m-HMPAO: a radiotoxicity study using the micronucleus assay. J Nucl Med 1992;33:1167-1174.
9. Merz T, Tatum J, Hirsch J. 99mTc labeled lymphocytes: a radiotoxicity study. J Nucl Med 1986;27:105-110.TK

10. Meignan M, Charpentier B, Wirquin E, Chavaudra J, Fries D, Galle P. Biological effects and irradiation dose induced in human lymphocytes in vitro by an intracellular radionuclide: ^{99m}Tc. Radiat Res 1983;94:263-279.

11. Bassano DA, McAfee JG. Cellular radiation doses of labeled neutrophils and platelets. J Nucl Med 1979;20:255-259.

12. Fourre C, Halpern S, Jeusset J, Clerc J, Fragu P. Significance of secondary ion mass spectrometry microscopy for technetium-99m mapping in leukocytes. J Nucl Med 1992;33:2162-2166.

13. Chisholm PM, Peters AM.The effect of indium-111 labeling on the recirculation of rat lymphocytes. In: Thakur ML, Gottschalk A, editors. Indium-111 labeled neutrophils, platelets, and lymphocytes. New York: Trivirum, 1980:205-208.

14. Wagstaff J. Lymphocyte migration studies in man. In: Thakur M, editor. Radiolabeled cellular blood elements (NATO ASI series). New York: Plenum Press; 1985:319-342.

15. Sprent J. Migratory properties and radiosensitivity of lymphocytes. In: Thakur M, editor. Radiolabeled cellular blood elements (NATO ASI series). New York: Plenum Press; 1985:31-50.

16. Thakur ML, Segal AW, Louis L, Welch MJ, Hopkins J, Peters TJ. Indium-111-labeled cellular blood components: mechanism of labeling and intracellular location in human neutrophils. J Nucl Med 1977;18:615-620.

17. Puncher MRB, Blower PJ. Frozen section microautoradiography in the study of radionuclide targeting: application to In-111-oxine labeled leukocytes. J Nucl Med 1995;36:499-505.

18. Davis HH, Senior RM, Griffin GL, Kuhn C. Indium-111-labeled human alveolar macrophages and monocytes: function and ultrastructure. J Immunol Methods 1980;36:99-107.

19. Costa DC, Lui D, Ell PJ. White cells radiolabelled with In-111 and Tc-99m - a study of relative sensitivity and in vivo viability. Nucl Med Commun 1988;9:725-731.

20. Puncher MRB, Blower PJ. Autoradiography and density gradient separation of Tc-99m-Exametazime (HMPAO) labelled leucocytes reveals selectivity for eosinophils. Eur J Nucl Med 1994;21:1175-1182.

21. Labriolle-Vaylet C, Colas-Linhart N, Petiet A, Bok B. Leucocytes marques a l' HMPAO- Tc-99m: etudes fonctionelles et microautoradiographiques. J Med Nucl Biophys 1990;14:137-141.

22. Hanna R, Braun T, Levendel A, Lomas F. Radiochemistry and biostability of autologous leucocytes labelled with Tc-99m-stannous colloid in whle blood. Eur J Nucl Med 1984;9:216-219.

23. Hanna R, Lomas F. Identification of factors affecting technetium-99m leucocyte labelling by phagocytic engulfment and development of an optimal technique. Eur J Nucl Med 1986;12:159-162.

24. Mock BH, English D. Leukocyte labeling with technetium-99m tin colloids. J Nucl Med 1987;28:1471-1477.

25. Puncher MRB, Blower PJ. Labelling of leucocytes with colloidal Tc-99m-SnF$_2$: an investigation of the labelling process by autoradiography. Eur J Nucl Med 1995;22:101-107.

26. Peters AM, Saverymuttu SH, Lavender JP. Granulocyte kinetics. In: Thakur M, editor. Radiolabeled cellular blood elements (NATO ASI series). New York: Plenum Press; 1985:285-303.

27. ten Berge RJM, Natarajan AT, Hardeman MR, van Royen EA, Schellekens PTA. Labeling with ^{111}In has detrimental effects on human lymphocytes: concise communication. J Nucl Med 1983;18:1012-1019.

28. Danpure HJ, Osman S. Radiolabelling human leucocytes and platelets for clinical studies. In: Theobald AE, editor. Radiopharmaceuticals: using radioactivecompounds in pharmaceutics and medicine. Chichester, UK: Ellis Horwood, 1989:65-79.

29. Frost P, Frost H. Recirculation of lymphocytes and the use of indium-111. J Nucl Med 1979;20:169.

CHAPTER 5

THE THORAX

Michael J. O'Doherty

Introduction

There are few conditions in humans that affect most people in the population at some time during their lives, lung inflammation/infection is such a problem. Airways inflammation or infection are a major cause of morbidity and accounts for a large number of visits of patients to their primary care physician. The inflammatory reaction is associated with marked vascular change including hyperaemia and vascular leakiness leading to interstitial oedema. These responses to noxious insults to the lung may lead to damage of the epithelium and due to excess production of mucous and cells to deal with the injury, blockage of airways may occur. The type of initiating injury often determines the type of cellular infiltrate and the response of the individual may be excessive leading to other problems in the lung. The response may affect the airflow and therefore delivery of oxygen and perhaps medication. Therapy to the lungs is often appropriately given via the airways by metered dose inhaler or nebulisers, the mode of this delivery can be studied using radionuclides but is beyond the scope of this chapter and has been reviewed recently [1]. The mechanisms behind the clearance of secretions associated with inflammatory and infective diseases are a further area where nuclear medicine techniques have contributed to the understanding of disease processes. Nuclear medicine studies can therefore contribute to the topic of inflammation and infection in the thorax in terms of understanding pathology, disease progression and management as well as investigating methods to improve therapy.

Infection and inflammation within the thorax is normally associated with either specific symptoms of breathlessness, cough, chest pain (pleuritic, pericarditic or musculoskeletal) or non-specific with fever, lethargy and confusion. The manner in which a patient presents determines the clinician's investigation strategy. The use of nuclear imaging in the thorax for inflammatory/infective disease is to provide diagnostic information to the clinician or at least confirm their suspicion as to the site needing to be treated or

81

P. H.Cox and J. R. Buscombe (eds.), The Imaging of Infection and Inflammation, 81–117.
© 1998 Kluwer Academic Publishers. Printed in the Netherlands.

biopsied. Other radionuclide investigations may provide an opportunity to follow a disease process sequentially or to monitor response to therapy.

Although morphologic imaging such as Computed Tomography (CT) or Magnetic Resonance Imaging (MRI) provide detailed anatomical information, they have a limited role in evaluating patients with long-term structural abnormalities or functional changes with little structural alteration. Subtle changes to the lung parenchyma having a large functional impact may not be visualised as a structural change. To utilise these modalities effectively a specific question needs to be asked and this may not always be clear in the clinician's mind.

The variety of problems caused by inflammation and infection within the thorax are determined by the structures within the thorax. The techniques used in the detection of inflammation/infection in these structures have been identified in other chapters and include Gallium-67, leucocyte imaging, labelled antibodies including antigranulocyte antibodies, polyclonal immunoglobulin and monoclonal antibodies specifically against Pneumocystis carinii pneumonia (PCP) and various bacteria. The only additional tests used in the thorax are the use of technetium diethylene triaminepentaacetic acid (DTPA) and the use of pyrophosphate or antimyosin antibodies which will be discussed. The measurement of clearance or transfer of ^{99m}Tc DTPA is related to the permeability of the lung epithelium to ^{99m}Tc DTPA and any process which causes disruption of the alveolar and respiratory bronchiole epithelium will increase this permeability. Lung ^{99m}Tc DTPA transfer (permeability, clearance) is measured by assessing the rate of loss of DTPA from the lung after it has been inhaled as an aerosol for 1 - 2 minutes, the particle size should be less than 1 micron. Data is acquired dynamically and the resultant time activity curves analysed to provide a clearance/transfer half time [2].

The investigation of thoracic inflammation and infection will be considered in this chapter by the structures within the thorax and limited to studies performed in human subjects. The areas that are discussed in other chapters e.g. bone infection are only considered here in terms of specific infections within the chest.

Extra Pulmonary Problems.

Skeletal System.

Infection and inflammation in the chest may affect the sternoclavicular joints, the sternum, the clavicles, the vertebrae and less commonly the ribs. Osteomyelitis can affect these areas after trauma, surgery or as a primary site. The most common problem within the ribs is a result of inflammation in costochondral joints. There are rare causes of multiple areas of increased uptake within ribs or of the clavicle which can be seen on conventional bone scanning which may be due to infection and should be questioned in the immunosuppressed patient. These multiple abnormalities in the immunosuppressed patient in the correct clinical setting may indicate bacillary angiomatosis [3]. Other abnormalities include discitis due to acute osteomyelitis or indeed due to tuberculosis, brucellosis etc.

A singular problem in the thorax is fever in a patient following a sternal split for cardiac bypass graft surgery. The bone scan is invariably positive and the question is whether there is infection present. Sternal wounds following bypass grafting can be investigated by ^{99m}Tc exametazime or ^{111}In labelled cells. Serry et al [4] reviewed 4,124 median sternotomies performed for cardiac surgery. Fifty patients had some form of complication of which 19 had septicaemia and mediastinal abscess in addition to the sternum infection. Therefore the mediastinum has to be viewed in this patient group. Salit et al [5] using gallium to evaluate patients with suspected sternal osteomyelitis found a sensitivity of 86% and specificity of 93% for osteomyelitis. By adding single photon emission tomography (SPET) the mediastinum can be evaluated as well. Cooper et al [6] investigated 29 patients to exclude deep sternal wound infection following coronary artery bypass grafting using ^{99m}Tc exametazime labelling and showed that intense uptake at 4 and 24 hours or increasing uptake between 4 and 24 hours was associated with deep sternal infection (100% sensitive; 89% specific). Superficial sternal infection was not reliably detected. Since the late images were superior to the early images it may be more appropriate to use ^{111}In labelled leucocytes rather than ^{99m}Tc to assess late changes, this study has not been performed. Leucocyte imaging is the most appropriate method to assess possible sternal osteomyelitis with additional mediastinal infection.

Heart and Great Vessels.
Pericarditis, myocarditis and cardiac transplant rejection.

Most causes of pericarditis and myocarditis are due to viral infection and more rarely due to bacterial, fungal and protozoal infection. The incidence of these diseases is increased in the immunosuppressed patient. Although the history and the clinical signs may strongly suggest the diagnosis, confirmation is sometimes required. Peri-myocarditis may be difficult to diagnose on the basis of the ECG or indeed echocardiography. Pericardial or myocardial pain may be investigated further by nuclear imaging. The utilisation of pyrophosphate, Gallium-67 or ^{111}In antimyosin antibody scanning may help (Fig.1).

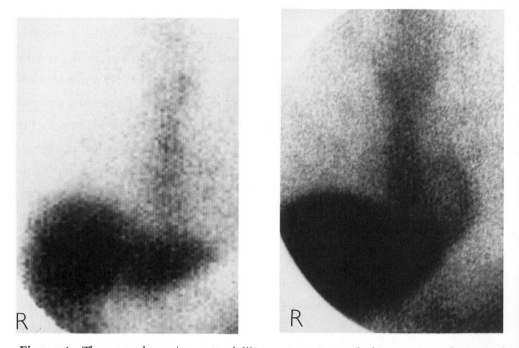

Figure 1. *The scans show a) a normal ^{111}In antimyosin antibody scan at 48 hours and diffuse uptake in the myocardium at 48 hours in a patient with a myocarditis.*

Cardiac problems associated with HIV include cardiomyopathy, myocarditis, Kaposi sarcoma, metastatic lymphoma, pericarditis and endocarditis. Unexpected increased accumulation of gallium-67 in the heart indicates further investigation is necessary; this appearance has been reported in myocarditis [7]. A normal scan however will not exclude a myocarditis. There are isolated case reports on the use of gallium-67 in Kawasaki's disease [8] and a report on the identification of associated myocarditis using ^{99m}Tc exametazime[9]. This latter paper examined 22 infants in the acute phase of Kawasaki's disease and 18 were thought to have myocarditis on the basis of clinical examination, ECG, echocardiogram. The uptake at 24 hours on the leucocyte scan identifed 18 cases of myocarditis whereas the gallium scan was only positive in one case.

Yasuda et al [10] demonstrated increased uptake of ^{111}In antimyosin antibody in patients with myocarditis, but a proportion of these patients had a negative biopsy. A question raised by this study was the magnitude of biopsy sampling error. The use of ^{111}In antimyosin Fab fragment in a large study of patients with suspected myocarditis showed a sensitivity of 83%, but a specificity of only 55% [11]. A proportion of these patients were followed up and 54% of those that had positive scans showed an improvement in their ejection fractions whereas those that had no uptake only 4 out of 22 had a marginal improvement in ejection fraction. The data suggested that endomyocardial biopsy is unlikely to confirm myocarditis in the presence of a normal antimyosin scan. Furthermore it may be concluded that the sampling error of the biopsy may be a major cause of the low specificity of the antimyosin scan.

In heart transplant patients the diffuse increased uptake of ^{111}In antimyosin antibody has been a useful monitor of acute rejection and a guide to those needing biopsy. The scan was positive in 52% of cases with histological rejection, but despite this low specificity it had a 100% sensitivity [12] and therefore may be useful in selection of patients for biopsy. Quantitation of uptake in patients followed up 1 year after transplant, identified those patients with moderate rejection [13]. Carrio et al [14] used quantitation (comparing the heart/lung ratios at 48 hours) in patients with heart transplants and found that the episodes of rejection were identified by the scan but that some scan positive patients did not have rejection confirmed on biopsy. One study challenges the concept that the anti-myosin scan is correct and biopsies are incorrect due to sampling; Obrador et al [15] looked at the uptake of antimyosin in 21 patients with dilated cardiomyopathy awaiting cardiac transplant. Fifteen patients had abnormal uptake and only 7 had an active myocarditis found in the heart that was removed at transplant surgery. It may still be argued that the histological examination did not include ultrastructural examination and thus minimal damage may have been missed.

The value of antimyosin antibody imaging is perhaps in the evaluation of patients with cardiac type pain or symptoms who do not have a clear diagnosis when the distinction between myocardial infarction and myocarditis is needed. Difficulty with scan interpretation can occasionally arise because of the slow clearance of the Fab fragment from the blood pool and the slow uptake in the myocardium, allowing misinterpretation of the diffuse blood pool activity as a myocarditis. New tracers have been developed to enhance this clearance from the blood pool [16].

Endocarditis.

The sensitivity of Gallium-67 scans in bacterial endocarditis is variable and may be influenced by the use of antibiotics and the site of the disease. Wiseman et al [17] reported positive scans in 6 out of 11 patients scanned at 72 hours, whereas Melvis et al [18] only found increased uptake in 2 out of 28 patients and neither of these identified the valve involved. The difference in the two studies was that the latter study had patients with predominantly right sided endocarditis and in all patients antibiotics has been started.

The use of a murine monoclonal ^{99m}Tc labelled anti NCA-95 antigranulocyte antibody BW 250/183 has been evaluated in 72 patients with suspected endocarditis [19]. Planar scintigraphy and SPET of the thorax were performed at approximately 24 hours. The technique demonstrated true positive scans in 26 patients and false positive in seven demonstrating a sensitivity of 79% and a specificity of 82%. Echocardiography had a sensitivity of 88% and specificity of 97%. The antibody scintigraphy was positive in four patients who had a negative echocardiogram. The repeat studies showed improvement in the scintigraphy paralleling the clinical improvement.

Although the use of SPET leucocyte imaging may have a role in detecting root abscesses it is likely that the mainstay of diagnosis of endocarditis will be the echocardiogram. It is difficult to understand why leucocytes or indeed gallium would localise in vegetations that are essentially intravascular, although interstitial abscesses at the valve roots would allow migration of cells. Whole body imaging detecting metastatic abscesses may however point to a diagnosis of endocarditis

Pleural Disease.

The use of leucocyte imaging in pleural disease is restricted. The diagnosis of pleural pathology usually depends on biopsy or aspiration. However coincidental finding of pleural uptake in patients in whom a source of a pyrexia is being sought is occasionally seen. Diffuse uptake of gallium around the pleura or leucocyte accumulation at a site of prior surgery may indicate a source of infection (fig.2). The difficult area of recurrence of malignant disease after lung resection can be confused with an empyema when ^{18}F-FDG is used as the tracer (fig.3).

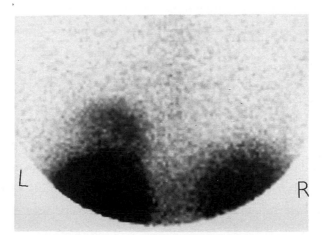

Figure 2. *The scan appearances show increased uptake of ^{111}In oxine labelled leucocytes in an empyema in the left lower chest.*

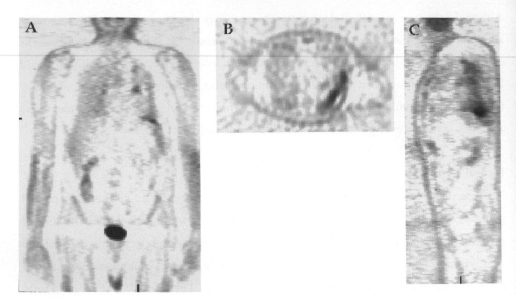

Figure 3. *A half body* ^{18}F *Fluorodeoxyglucose PET scan showing A) coronal B) transaxial and C) sagittal cuts through the left lower lobe empyema and regional hilar lymph node accumulation of DFG. This presents potential difficulty in distinguishing a pleural carcinoma and a hilar metastasis.*

Lymph node disease.

Lymph nodes in the hila, mediastinum and the subcarinal structures may demonstrate reactive change associated with infection within the lung or direct involvement in granulomatous processes e.g. sarcoidosis or mycobacterial infections. Lymphadenopathy can be assessed using Gallium-67, ^{18}F-fluorodeoxyglucose (FDG) or the combination of Thallium-201 and Gallium-67 to assess whether disease is inflammatory or malignant in nature. Discussion about the distinction between tumour and inflammation is beyond the scope of this chapter. Assessment of sarcoidosis may include high uptake in the mediastinum and hilum which may be associated with uptake in the parenchymal tissue and is discussed below under parenchymal lung disease. The utility of these diagnostic agents are discussed below. The agents are not normally used to assess known lymphadenopathy, but rather lymphadenopathy is found during whole body assessment of patients with a pyrexia of unknown origin or suspected malignancy.

Pulmonary disease.

The lung parenchyma provides an enormous exposed surface to the air. Approximately 20,000 litres of air pass over the epithelial surfaces of the lung per 24 hours. These air exchanges allow particles of bacteria, viruses, antigens and various chemicals to come into direct contact with the lung surface and potentially irritate or cause severe disease. These disease processes can be evaluated by a number of imaging techniques. A variety of diseases e.g. collagen diseases have secondary efects on the lung and these may result in problems for the patient.

Inflammatory lung disease.

Alveolar and interstitial diseases.

This group of patients tend to have diffuse disease affecting both lungs. Normally the patient will present with breathlessness, a cough and possibly fever, with the chest radiograph often abnormal although not invariably. An indication of the cause of the underlying disease may be given by the patient's occupation, hobbies, medication or by a history of immunosuppression related to the human immunodeficiency virus (HIV) or drug therapy. Investigations often do not involve nuclear medicine although the tests that can be offered may be used in monitoring disease or at least indicating the most affected areas of the lung for biopsy.

Extrinsic allergic alveolitis.

There are a number of possible causes of this condition but the histological change in the subacute phase is that of non-caseating granulomata with oedema and thickening of the alveolar walls. This disruption of the alveolar membrane by cell infiltrates has been monitored using the technique of lung ^{99m}Tc DTPA clearance/transfer and has been shown to be abnormal in at least one cause of the condition "pigeon fanciers" lung [20]. The clearance rate is increased in this condition, and appears to be related to the amount of antibody in the blood since those patients with high levels of antibody had increased clearance and those patients with antigen exposure but without an antibody response had faster times than normal controls but not as fast as those with antibody. The clearance rates were increased when conventional pulmonary function test were normal.

Cryptogenic fibrosing alveolitis

There are a variety of disease processes that affect the alveolar regions of the lung which include cryptogenic fibrosing alveolitis, connective tissue diseases [21], radiation pneumonitis and drug induced alveolitis [22] as well as infection. All of these conditions affect the transfer of ^{99m}Tc DTPA as a marker of the inflammatory damage to the lung (figs.4,5). Serial measurements of ^{99m}Tc DTPA clearance have been made to follow response to therapy in cryptogenic fibrosing alveolitis [23,24].

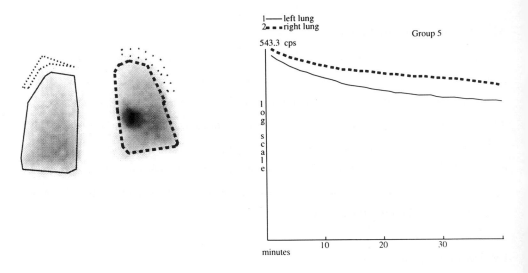

Figure 4.[99m] *Tc DTPA transfer curves in bleomycin induced alveolitis in a patient with lymphoma. The transfer times are biphasic (at least biexponential); the first component half times for the left lung were 3 min and for the right lung 3.5 min.*

Fibrosing alveolitis is characterised by the infiltration of the lung parenchyma with inflammatory cells that may lead to progressive fibrosis. The degree and distribution of the inflammation and fibrosis can be assessed by open lung biopsy; bronchoalveolar lavage can assess the amount of inflammation but not the relative amounts of fibrosis and inflammation, similarly pulmonary function tests cannot discriminate. Labrune et al [23] demonstrated a positive correlation between the rate of DTPA clearance and alveolar lymphocytosis which negatively correlated with vital capacity. They also demonstrated that the DTPA clearance rate decreased when patients responded to corticosteroids but the rate did not return to normal.

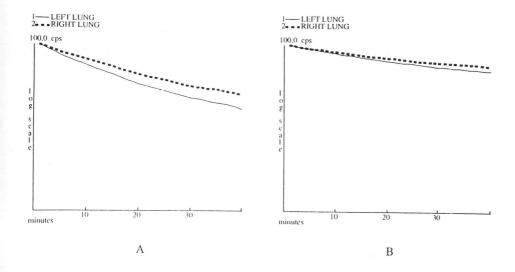

A   B

Figure 5. [99m] *Tc DTPA transfer curves in fibrosing aveolitis A) pre and B) post treatment with steroids. The curves are presented as a plot of lung activity against time. There is an improvement in the transfer times as seen by a decrease in the slope of the time activity curves*

The persistent increase in the clearance of DTPA may be a result of the stretching of lung units by fibrosis. The test represents a potential method for documenting response to steroids allowing follow up as they are reduced. Uh et al [25] examined the clearance of ^{99m}Tc DTPA in patients with diffuse infiltrative lung disease (DILD) and found that for patients with DILD the T½ was significantly shorter in all lobes than normal controls, but that patients with early stage disease had longer times than those with late disease in the upper and middle lobes. There was however overlap between the normal range and those patients with disease, such that it was difficult to use the test to identify those patients with disease and normal carbon monoxide transfer values. Thus it is unlikely to be a diagnostic test but may be used to monitor therapy and relapse.

Gallium-67 scanning has been performed in a variety of diffuse infiltrative lung conditions. These include sarcoidosis (described below), idiopathic fibrosing alveolitis [26,27,28], drug toxicity [29,30], pneumoconiosis [31], pneumocystis carinii pneumonia (see below) and a variety of other conditions including diffuse acute bacterial and viral pneumonitis, carcinomatosis and post irradiation [32]. Usually the diffuse abnormality on the gallium scan suggests the need for further investigation or depending on the clinical situation the likely disease process. In fibrosing alveolitis gallium scanning has been used to stage the disease. A good correlation has been reported between disease activity on transbronchial biopsy and gallium uptake [26]. The closest correlation however was found with the neutrophil content of bronchoalveolar lavage fluid and not the lymphocyte count which is surprising in view of the cellular response in the interstitium.

Drug and radiation induced pneumonitis.

A variety of drugs can cause a pneumonitis, the most common is bleomycin induced toxicity. Other drug causes are far less common but amiodarone toxicity can present a problem in distinguishing an alveolitis from interstitial pulmonary oedema due to heart failure, since the drug is used in patients with cardiac disease. The differential diagnosis is therefore between congestive cardiac failure and amiodarone pneumonitis. Since cardiac failure does not alter the alveolar-capillary interface the transfer of DTPA in these conditions is normal [33] then this test should be able to separate cardiogenic from an alveolitic cause of breathlessness. Terra-Filho et al [34] demonstrated that the clearance half times were faster than normal non-smokers and patients on amiodarone but with no respiratory problems. The technique of DTPA clearance was more sensitive than spirometry in detecting this condition. It would however not have distinguished smokers who had pneumonitis. Further abnormalities have been reported in the inflammatory response due to "crack" use with increased clearance detected [22]. O'Doherty et al [35] reported a differential effect on pulmonary clearance throughout the lungs of patients with haematological malignancy trated with a variety of cytotoxic drugs with the effect greater at the base of the lung than the apex. The postulate was that this effect was distributed according to the blood flow and thus the concentration of the drug delivery to the lung, but no biopsy proof for this was available.

Gallium scans are also abnormal in acute inflammation associated with drug induce pneumonitis or radiation induced pneumonitis [29,30]. These changes present problems in distinguishing drug induced damage from diffuse uptake due to infection.

Connective tissue disorders affecting the lung.

All connective tissue diseases can potentially affect the lung. Usually the inflammatory process affects the bases more than the apices of the lung. This has been demonstrated in early publications on ^{99m}Tc DTPA clearance [21]. Chopra et al [36] studied a group of patients with systemic sclerosis and found that the ^{99m}Tc DTPA clearance from the lung was much faster in the affected lower zones. Gallium-67 has been reported to have increased uptake in the lungs of patients with pulmonary involvement with systemic lupus erythematosis [37] and one would expect similar increased uptake to be observed with acute changes associated with rheumatoid arthritis and polyarteritis nodosa. However no uptake was seen in patients with scleroderma or chronic rheumatoid lung [37]. This would be consistent with fibrosis without inflammation in these lesions.

Adult respiratory distress syndrome.

Widespread severe inflammation associated with the adult respiratory distress syndrome has been evaluated with lung permeability measurements both of the vascular and the epithelial surfaces. These techniques reflect the structural damage that can be done to the membranes of the lung. Lung ^{99m}Tc DTPA transfer has been shown to have fast transfer rates [33], the amount of damage to the endothelium has also been shown to be severe using ^{113m}In transferrin accumulation within the lung [38]. Braude S. et al [39] demonstrated a correlation between ^{99m}Tc DTPA transfer and the ^{113m}In transferrin measurement in patients with adult respiratory distress syndrome. This illustrates that the movement of molecules from the vascular space to the airspace can give comparable results to the movement from the airspace to the vascular space. This degree of structural damage has also been shown using PET techniques in humans [40,41] and dogs [42,43] by showing the changes in blood flow using ^{15}O H_2O, protein flux ^{68}Ga transferrin and blood volume ^{15}O CO measurements. The degree of inflammation and damage can be shown in infants with respiratory distress syndrome using ^{99m}Tc DTPA [44]. The question perhaps is why bother since the damage is known from the blood gases and the CXR. The measurements used with PET are the transcapillary escape rate and the normalised slope index. These measurements potentially provide a marker of acute lung injury and a means of separating cardiogenic pulmonary oedema from noncardiogenic causes. The marker may also provide an insight into the mechanism and a means of predicting patients who will respond and recover or at least enable an evaluation of therapy options.

Granulomatous diseases of the Lung.

There are a variety of granulomatous disease that affect the lung including miliary tuberculosis, sarcoidosis and talc granulomatosis in intravenous drug use [32]. Gallium-67 scanning has been demonstrated to have increased uptake in these. The use of scanning is to define the extent of disease and the disease activity. The most studied disease process is pulmonary sarcoidosis.

Sarcoid.

Sarcoidosis is a multisystem inflammatory granulomatous disease which predominantly presents as pulmonary disease but can affect almost any organ. The presenting features in the lung are either pulmonary infiltrates or hilar and mediastinal lymphadenopathy, the chest radiograph however is highly insensitive and up to 60% of patients with granulomas in the parenchyma may have a normal chest radiograph. The differential diagnosis with the predominant hilar and mediastinal adenopathy is between lymphoma and sarcoidosis. The scales are tipped in favour of sarcoid by the ethnic origin of the patient. The predominant radionuclide is the assessment of sarcoidosis is Gallium-67 which shows a diffuse uptake in the lung in parenchymal sarcoid and intense uptake in the mediastinum and the hilum when these nodes are involved (fig.6,7).

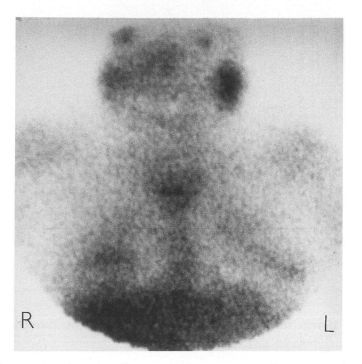

Figure 6. *An anterior thoracic gallium scan, the appearances show increased uptake in the parotid glands and low grade diffuse increased uptake in the lungs of a patient with predominant parenchymal sarcoid.*

The degree of lung uptake relates to disease activity [27]. The uptake has been described as the "lambda" distribution which has been found to be helpful particularly when associated with lachrymal, parotid and nasal uptake ("panda" pattern) in determining that the uptake is due to sarcoidosis [45,46]. Gallium-67 imaging is seen as a method of following the activity of disease in response to therapy [47,48]. Quantitation has been attempted using Gallium-67 to assess response of diffuse parenchymal uptake to therapy [49]. The other technique used to assess active sarcoid is the ^{99m}Tc DTPA transfer as a non-specific indicator of disease activity (see above).

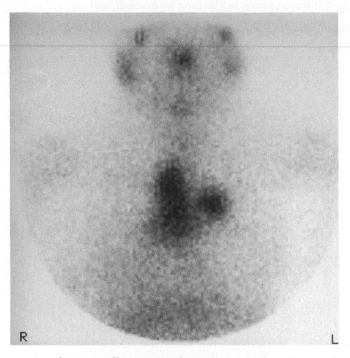

R   L

Figure 7. *An anterior thoracic gallium scan, the appearances show increased uptake in the hila and mediastinal lymph nodes in a patient with sarcoidosis*

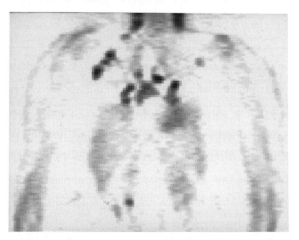

Figure 8. *A ¹⁸F FDG PET study in a patient with pulmonary sarcoidosis. The coronal cut shows uptake in the mediastinum, hilae, axillary and supraclavicular lymph nodes.*

^{18}F-FDG uptake has been documented in sarcoidosis (fig.8) due to the non-specific nature of FDG uptake in inflammation [50]. This uptake was demonstrated in lymph nodes [50] and has been demonstrated in the lung parenchyma [51]. Brudin et al [52] measured the regional glucose metabolism per gram of lung tissue using PET and found that the abnormal levels returned to normal during treatment with steroids. This improvement was similar to the change in angiotensin converting enzyme levels and was thought to reflect "disease activity". In vitro, FDG has been shown to be taken up by leucocytes, lymphocytes and macrophages [53] and therefore it is a non-specific tracer.

Lung permeability is also increased in pulmonary sarcoidosis. The increase in ^{99m}Tc DTPA flux across the epithelial membrane of the lung has been observed in Type I, II and III pulmonary sarcoidosis [54,55,56]. The transfer increases with deterioration in pulmonary function as well as decreasing with response to treatment with steroids [54]. The transfer is thought to be related to the degree of inflammation associated with the sarcoidosis, but the rate of transfer has no definite relationship to the serum angiotensin converting enzyme levels or to the lymphocyte amounts in bronchoalveolar lavage fluid.

Other imaging in granulomatous diseases in addition to sarcoidosis has been demonstrated with ^{111}In octreotide [57]. The abnormal uptake occurred in lung parenchyma as well as lymph nodes. This was more sensitive than radiological imaging but no comparison was made with Gallium-67 which would have been of greater interest. The method does appear to document response to treatment, although in this study only five patients were followed, in two the scans became negative and three remained positive with apparent failure of response to therapy by other parameters. Other approaches to the imaging of sarcoidosis are being developed with the use of macrophage targeted glycolipepetide JOO1 [58], their usefulness remains to be seen.

Wegeners granulomatosis.

Patients with systemic vasculitis have been shown to have increased margination of leucocytes within the lung [59] and in the case of Wegeners granulomatosis have been shown to have focal nasal uptake [59] in addition to focal uptake within the lung parenchyma [60].

Two patients with Wegeners granulomatosis have had positive uptake with ^{111}In octreotide visualised in the lung [57].

Mycobacterial infections.

Mycobacterial infections have had a resurgence with the onset of HIV infection. The use of Gallium-67 imaging in mycobacterium tuberculosis identifies the sites of infection (Fig.9) and has been shown to have a diffuse uptake in miliary tuberculosis [61].

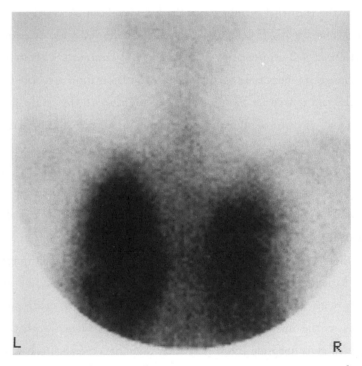

Figure 9. *The posterior thoracic gallium scan appearances in a patient with miliary mycobacterium tuberculosis. Diffuse uptake is demonstrated throughout both of the lungs*

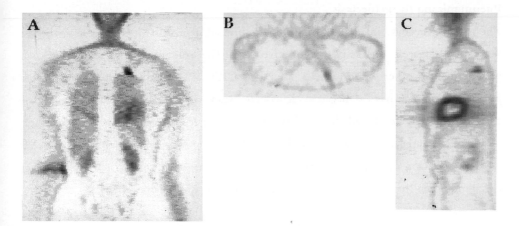

Figure 10. *A ^{18}F FDG scan in a patient with left upper lobe opacity and suspicious cells on needle aspiration. The lesion has a high uptake on FDG uptake seen on the coronal (A), transaxial (B) and the sagittal (C) cuts, despite the high uptake this was not a carcinoma but was shown to be mycobacterium tuberculosis.*

In the population of patients that tend to have tuberculosis, consideration has to be given to the fact that talc granulomatosis will also lead to a diffuse increased uptake [32]. Increased uptake of gallium in the chest may localise the atypical mycobacterial infections, which may also be found in lymph nodes as well as soft tissue (see below in the section on immunosuppression). Abnormal uptake may also be seen with ^{111}In octreotide imaging [57].

PET imaging has also been shown to be abnormal with tuberculosis and may lead to confusion in peripheral lesions within the lung (Fig.10). These lesions may have high standardised uptake values. Patz et al [62] reported high FDG uptake in tuberculosis and fungal infections in the lung. The identification of such abnormalities may direct the clinician to the correct area to biopsy. The advantage over gallium imaging is the capability of same day imaging with higher resolution and in the future the opportunity to register the PET image to the CT to allow precise anatomical definition of the abnormality.

Pneumoniaand Bronchiectasis.

The role of leucocyte imaging in the thorax is limited. It may be used to assess whether bronchiectatic areas are active or inactive [63]. The role in straight forward lobar pneumonia or other abnormalities seen on CXR is severely limited since lobar pneumonia often has a negative leucocyte scan, presumably because once the consolidation has developed there is little turnover of leucocytes in the abnormal area [64]. The potential is in a abnormal chest with chronic abnormalities on CT or CXR where a suspicion of disease activity is raised and needle aspiration or surgical drainage is required then the focus of infection may be localised using leucocytes.

Detection of Inflammation/Infection in the lung of immunosuppressed Patients.

The lung is the most commonly affected organ in the immunocompromised host and mortality is often high. Therefore a fever and a new lung symptom or sign presents an urgent clinical problem. There are a wide variety of possible causes of fever in the immunocompromised patient which tends to confound the choice of empirical therapy. The patients are often debilitated from the underlyeing disease and therefore invasive investigations are hazardous. The question is therefore does nuclear medicine have anything to offer in this patient population? There are differences which depend on he cause of the immunosuppressed state. For example if the patient is suppressed by chemotherapy compared with HIV disease then the underlying infection causing the pyrexia will be different and also is likely to have a different urgency with regards to investigation. Often the HIV patient with a fever and respiratory symptoms can be investigated in a little more slowly than the former group who may become unwell very quickly. The frequency of certain infections vary between the HIV positive patients and the iatrogenic group, transplanted patients have a higher incidence of cytomegalovirus (CMV) infection [65], whereas HIV positive patients have a higher incidence of PCP and bacterial infections such as streptococcus pneumoniae, pseudomonas aerogenosa and mycobacteria. Fungal infections may occur in either group.

In the patient who is neutropenic due to chemotherapy the investigation clinician is likely to want an instant test to demonstrate the type of abnormality and the distribution of the abnormality to direct further investigation. The use of ^{99m}Tc DTPA clearance can demonstrate the location of the main ventilatory abnormality if there is a focal problem before the chest radiograph changes or the clearance/transfer times may indicate the presence of a pneumonitis. Thus in renal transplant patients PCP has a rapid transfer time for DTPA [66] but these changes would also occur with CMV infection which is common in transplant patients, therefore the test is used to direct investigation away from a possible cause of fluid overload or a bacterial pneumonia towards a definitive invasive test, transbronchial biopsy, or an urgent induced sputum examination. The alternative tests would be Gallium-67 scanning which has a variable uptake in CMV and therefore a variable sensitivity [67,68]. ^{111}In leucocyte scans have also been shown to be positive in CMV pneumonitis [69]. Although it may be stated that gallium has a lower uptake in CMV than PCP, the unfortunate truth is that this fact is unhelpful in the individual since the uptake of gallium in PCP is so variable. The most discriminatory role for gallium and ^{99m}Tc DTPA is in the patient with a normal chest radiograph. The DTPA scan in patients on chemotherapy is of less diagnostic value since agents such as bleomycin will also produce a pneumonitis and therefore although the cause of the breathlessness is identified as a pneumonitis the differential is far greater than in HIV positive patients.

With the increasing use of immunosuppressants in a variety of diseases the clinician has to be aware of the potential disease processes affecting the lungs and the effect of the various immunosuppressants on the lungs. Patients are more susceptible to a range of bacterial, fungal and viral illnesses. The use of leucocytes labelled with either ^{99m}Tc exametazime or ^{111}In oxine or tropolone can be effected using donor leucocytes (Fig.11) rather than autologous cells in patients who are HIV positive [70], or by using agents that can be labelled from manufacturers kits e.g. antigranulocyte antibodies, polyclonal antibodies or human immunoglobulin IgG. Usually leucocyte imaging is best applied to infections which are outside the chest [71] although disease may be localised coincidentally while looking elsewhere. The use of an antigranulocyte antibody to try and detect a variety of lung infections in HIV positive patients has proven to be unsuccessful, confirming the fact that this method should not be used for respiratory infections [72]. The technique may be unsuccessful for a number of reasons and may be related to few neutrophils present or the fact that the patients own neutrophils were not functioning adequately. An alternative non-specific method of examining inflammation in the lung is to use aerosolised ^{99m}Tc DTPA as a reflection of lung permeability.

Often the clinician wants to know whether the source of the temperature is in the chest or elsewhere and then decide on a course of investigation as rapidly as possible or institute empirical therapy. The nuclear physician has to be aware of the differential diagnosis of various tests when they show abnormalities within the lung especially in this era of HIV diseases when the range of infections, tumours etc. affecting young men and women are increased.

Gallium has been the preferred agent to assess the thorax since it allows visualisation of the lung parenchyma, soft tissues, heart and lymph nodes. Scans can be performed as early as 4 hours and as late as 7 days after the injection of 150 - 400 MBq of Gallium-67. Late imaging may be useful in detecting mediastinal disease with tomography after injection of 400 MBq of Gallium-67. Unless a department has gallium in stock the imaging procedure may be delayed by several days, therefore to improve the efficiency in giving the clinician a diagnosis, protocols for early imaging and quantifying lung/liver count rate ratios at 4 hours following injection have been suggested [73]. These ratios were similar at 4,24, 48 en 72 hours in patients with PCP however it is likely this technique could be unreliable in those patients with disease of the liver where the uptake may be very low, for example in patients with hepatitis B or C disease, a common problem in this patient group (Fig.11).

The most common infection in patients with HIV infection is PCP although this is slowly changing. The classical appearance of a Gallium-67 scan in PCP is diffuse uptake in both lungs with a negative cardiac silhouette [74,75] but a variety of scan appearances can be seen [76,77]. Uptake in the lung can be graded between 0 (normal) and 4, by comparing the uptake in the lung to that in the liver and bone marrow, if this accumulation is less than (grade 2), equal to (grade 3) or higher (grade 4) than that

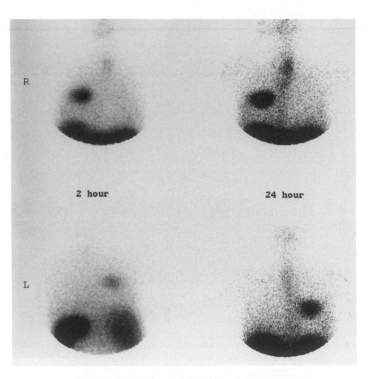

Figure 11. *A donor* ^{111}In *leucocyte scan in a HIV positive patient with a pseudomonas aerogenosa chest infection. The high accumulation of leucocytes is clearly seen on the 2 and 24 hour images*

in the liver and is diffuse, a confident diagnosis of diffuse lung disease can be made and the probability of this being due to PCP is high in HIV positive patients (Fig.12). If it is higher than normal but just less than the rib uptake (grade 1) this is equivocal uptake. However, in other immunosuppressed patients this will not be the case since cytomegalovirus infection or drug toxicity may be more prevalent. Low uptake in the context of an abnormal chest radiograph often carries a worse prognosis [74]. The sensivity and specificity of ^{67}Ga in PCP are 80 - 90% and 50 - 74% respectively [78], rising to 100% in those HIV positive patients with a normal chest X-ray [79]. An important point is that the negative predictive value for pulmonary pathology is high

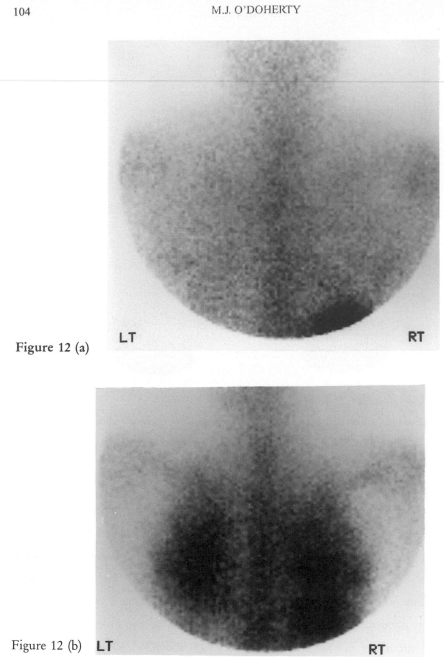

Figure 12 (a)

Figure 12 (b)

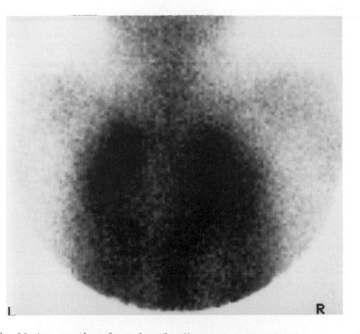

Figure 12.(c) *Various grades of uptake of gallium in patients with pneumocystis carinii pneumonia. Posterior scans are shown, the first A) has normal gallium distribution, the second B) has uptake which is slightly lower than liver uptake, the third C) has higher uptake in the lung than the liver.*

91%) [80] when both the CXR and the gallium scans are normal. The distribution of Gallium-67 within the chest in HIV positive patients may point to the pathology present. Bilateral upper lobe uptake can occur with PCP in patients treated with nebulised pentamidine [81], but this may also be seen in patients with mycobacterial infection. Similarly diffuse uptake may be seen with lymphocytic pneumonitis [82], non-specific pneumonitis [83] or miliary mycobacterial infection or probably cryptococcal infections.

Bacterial pneumonias tend to show focal accumulation in either a lobar or multilobar distribution with gallium imaging (Fig.13). If accumulation is focal in the lung and/or is associated with bone involvement, then atypical fungal infection or lymphoma should be considered in the differential diagnosis. Accumulation of gallium in regional lymph nodes in HIV positive patients within the chest is consistent with lymphoma, mycobacterium avium intracellulare, persistent generalised lymphadenopathy, pneumocystis carinii infection or other infective processes.

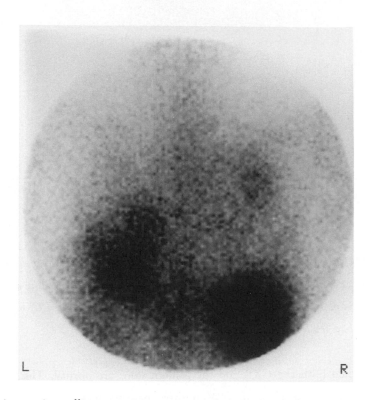

Figure 13. *A posterior gallium scan in a patient with a streptococcal pneumoniae infection. The scan shows the multiple foci of uptake of gallium in the left lower lobe and the right upper lobe*

The use of antibodies for the localisation of infection and inflammation has an advantage over leucocyte imaging because preparations are available in kit form and do not require handling of blood. This had a major advantage in HIV positive patients or those with neutropenia. The disadvantage of using Indium-111 as the radionuclide is that it is not produced on site and therefore has to be ordered especially for the labelling procedure. Animal and human studies have shown localisation of ^{111}In polyclonal antibodies (^{111}In HIgG) in lungs infected with PCP [84,85,86]. Imaging with ^{111}In and

[99mTc] HIgG has been studied [87,88]. It was found that HIgG had a superior sensitivity and specificity compared with [99mTc] HIgG, which was thought to be due to the later imaging at 48 hours with [111In] HIgG. This allowed a greater clearance of HIgG from the blood pool. The pattern of uptake was diffuse with PCP and focal with bacterial infections. A recent study by Prvulovich et al [72] using antigranulocyte antibody imaging demonstrated the lack of localisation of infection within the chest, and poor localisation of infection elsewhere. This raises the question as to whether the neutropenic individual has sufficient labelling to localise or whether the neurophils are capable of functioning adequately in severe HIV disease. The technique may be suitable in immunosuppressed individuals from other causes.

Monoclonal antibody imaging, using a Fab' fragment raised in mice against pneumocystis carinii labelled with [99mTc], has been performed in HIV antibody positive patients and raises the possibility of a more specific test for PCP [89]. The 24 hour images provided the most reliable results. Only sixteen patients were studied with a presumptive or definite diagnosis of PCP, most had very abnormal chest radiographs. In this selected population the sensitivity and specificity were 85.7 and 86.7%. The technique raises the interesting possibility of its use in extrapulmonary disease detection but has not addressed the more relevant issues of whether uptake occurs in the lungs of patients with mild disease or normal chest radiographs. The study by Goldenberg et al [89] does indicate that therapy for PCP can be given without affecting the result since images were positive even when performed 28 days after the initiation of PCP treatment. This suggests that the test will be of little help in follow up studies.

Most of the above studies cannot be performed immediately on patients and therefore are unable to give a result on the same day. In patients with HIV infection who have a cough, breathlessness and a fever the question is normally: does the patient have PCP? Lung [99mTc] DTPA transfer can give an answer to this question or at least indicate whether the patient has pulmonary pathology. The technique has been investigated in PCP and other lung infections by a number of groups [1,90-94], all have documented a rapid transfer or clearance time. Our own studies show that in an alveolitis the appearance of the curve is biphasic, with a rapid first component (half-time < 4 minutes[12.5%/minute]) (Fig.14). The most likely cause of an alveolitis and hence the biphasic pattern (in HIV positive patients) is still PCP, but other causes of this pattern include CMV infection, lymphocytic interstitial pneumonitis and non-specific interstitial pneumonitis.

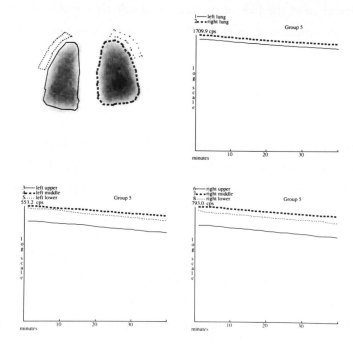

Figure 14 (a)

The test has a high sensitivity and specificity in this patient population for PCP, but false negative results may occur [92]. Occasionally a biphasic curve can be found in heavy smokers with HIV infection in the absence of an alveolitis and therefore it is suggested that baseline scans are performed in all smokers (authors experience). Transfer times are not biphasic in other bacterial infections (with the exception of Legionella pneumophila) [91]. Rosso et al [90] have demonstrated that the ^{99m}Tc DTPA technique has a higher sensitivity than gallium scanning (92%) compared with 72%) for infectious pulmonary complications [90]. This difference is more marked for patients with normal chest radiographs and normal blood gases. A normal chest radiograph and a normal DTPA clearance virtually exclude pulmonary infection/inflammation requiring therapy. A recent review of ^{99m}Tc DTPA transfer in HIV positive patients has outlined an

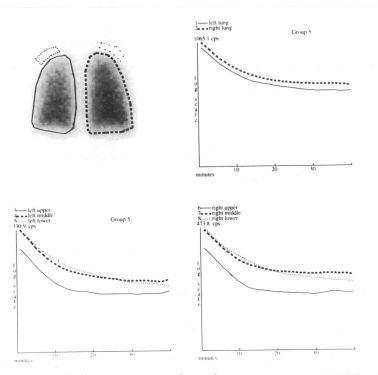

Figure 14 (a and b) *^{99m}Tc DTPA transfer study in an asymptomatic HIV positive patient and a patient with pneumocystis carinii pneumonia (PCP). The curves show A) a monoexponential pattern in the asymptomatic patient and B) a biphasic pattern when the patient developed PCP in all lung regions as well as the whole lung. The initial deposition of the aerosol is also shown.*

algorithm for its use in HIV infection [95]. This will cintinue to be of use only while PCP is the most common cause of an alveolitis in HIV positive patients.

A more recent development, Pertechnegas (which is generated from Technegas by the addition of oxygen) has been used to assess patients with HIV infection and respiratory symptoms [96]. This imaging technique appears to convey little advantage over ^{99m}Tc DTPA.

FDG PET scanning has also been used in the evaluation of HIV positive patients [97]. It is apparent that although the scan is expensive there are a number of advantages. The ability to evaluate the whole patient from the brain to the toes is a valuable asset but in particular the scan can assess the mediastinal nodes for increased uptake to direct further investigation. The results of such a study are available the same day and it is possible that quantitative data will be able to discriminate inflammatory change from infection and malignancy.

This method of scanning saves patient visitis to the department, can hasten patient investigation as an inpatient and may therefore save costs. These latter statements are currently speculative and need to be explored further.

Heart-Lung transplants.

With heart lung transplantation the problems associated with inflammation are infection and rejection. Early reports suggested that conventional ventilation perfusion scans performed on a quantitative basis could detect early rejection [98]. An inhomogeneous perfusion scan develops with the onset of rejection and that there is gradual reduction in blood flow to the affected lung with time. Skeens et al [99] however found that the appearance of cytolytic lymphocytes in bronchoalveolar lavage fluid was more sensitive than the quantitative perfusion scan. A further method of investigating rejection has been the use of ^{99m}Tc DTPA clearance [100]. This is more rapid in patients with lung transplants (2.62±0.25%/min) compared to nonsmoking controls (1.2±0.12%/min) and during rejection this clearance is more rapid (3.65±0.41%). The sensitivity and specificity of the measurement was 69 and 82% respectively whereas the use of FEV_1 had a sensitivity of 45% and specificity of 85%. These data suggest the technique may be a very simple method of monitoring this patient group, with biopsy if the clearance is increasing. Other pathology such as CMV and PCP would give similar changes to the clearance however.

Conclusion.

The thorax is an area of the body which is particularly suitable to assessment with nuclear imaging. The multifunctional roles of the lung in terms of gas exchange, drug metabolism present an area of interest for the delivery and absorption of drugs, the management of secretions and the maintenance of fluid balance across the vascular and epithelial surfaces. The increased use of cytotoxic drugs for cancer and for organ transplants increase the importance of noninvasive methods to localise sites of infection and inflammation. The areas of proven use are the investigation of mediastinal infection using ^{99m}Tc exametazime, mediastinal node inflammation with Gallium-67 and the assessment of parenchymal lung disease using Gallium-67 and ^{99m}Tc DTPA scanning. Both Gallium-67 and ^{99m}Tc DTPA can be used to monitor therapy and have been shown to predict improvement in the patients clinical condition e.g. sarcoidosis or response to PCP therapy in HIV positive patients. There is no clear role for imaging in endocarditis although it is possible that the use of antigranulocyte antibody imaging may have a selective role in assessing response to treatment in some patients. Myocardial imaging with antimyosin antibodies has a limited role in patients who are considered for endomyocardial biopsy since a negative scan in rejection and those suspected of having myocarditis makes the chance of obtaining a positive biopsy result very low.

The other areas of possible benefit in inflammation and infection are in the assessment of drug delivery to the lungs. This is achieved by direct labelling of drugs or indirect labelling of nebuliser solutions, thus assessing in semiquantitative terms delivery to areas of the lung. Other areas to be explored are the distribution of receptors within the lung e.g. β receptors and angiotensin converting enzyme and steroid sites using PET radionuclides. Further research on the capillary - alveolar interface may allow subgrouping of patients with ARDS into groups that require differing therapeutic strategies.

The number of days lost from work by adults due to respiratory and myocardial disease requires continued efforts to be made to evaluate investigative strategies within the thorax which will enable quick diagnosis and selection of the appropriate therapeutic intervention.

References

1. O'Doherty MJ, Miller RF. Aerosols for therapy and diagnosis. Eur J Nucl Med 1993;20 (12), 1201-1213.

2. O'Doherty MJ, Page CJ, Bradbeer CS et al. Alveolar permeability in HIG patients with pneumocystis carinii pneumonia. Genitourin Med 1987; 63:268-270.

3. Baron AL, Steinbach LS, Leboit PE, Mills CM, Gee JH, Berger TG. Osteolytic lesions of bacillary angiomatosis in HIV infection: radiologic differentiation from AIDS-related Kaposi sarcoma. Radiology 1990; 177: 77-81.

4. Serry C, Bleck PC, Javid H et al. Sternal wound complications. J Thorax Cardiovasc Surg 1980; 80:861-867.

5. Salit IE, Detsky AS, Simor AE et al. Gallium-67 scanning in the diagnosis of postoperative sternal osteomyelitis: concise communication. J Nucl Med 1983; 24: 1001-1004.

6. Cooper JA, Elmendorf SL, Teixeira III JP, McCandless BK, Foster ED. Diagnosis of sternal wound infection by technetium-99m-leucocyte imaging. J Nucl Med 1992; 33:59-65.

7. Cregler LL, Sosa I, Ducey S, Abbey S. Myopericarditis in acquired immunodeficiency syndrome diagnosed by gallium scintigraphy. J Nat Med Assoc. 1990; 82:511-513.

8. Sty JR, Chusid MJ, Dorrington A, Ga-67 imaging: Kawasaki disease. Clin Nucl Med 1981; 6:112-113.

9. Kao CH, Hsieh KS, Wang Yl et al. Comparison of 99mTc HMPAO-labelled white blood cells and 67 Ga citrate scans to detect myocarditis in the acute phase of Kawasaki disease. Nucl Med Commun 1995; 12:951-958.

10. Yasuda T. Palcios IF, Dec GW et al. Indium-111-monoclonal antimyosin antibody imaging in the diagnosis of acute myocarditis. Circulation 1987; 76:306-311.

11. Dec GW, Palacios I, Yasuda et al. Antimyosin antibody cardiac imaging: its role in the diagnosis of myocarditis. J A C C 1990; 16:97-104.

12. Frist W. Yasuda T. Segall G et al. Noninvasive detection of human cardiac transplant rejection with indium-111 antimyosin (Fab) imaging. Circulation 1987; 76:V81-V85.

13. Ballester-Rodes M, Carrio-Gasset I, Abadal-Berini L et al. Patterns of evolution of myocyte damage after human heart transplantation detected by indium-111 monoclonal antimyosin. Am J Cardiol 1988; 62:623-627.

14. Carrio I, Berna L, Ballester M et al. Indium-111 antimyosin scintigraphy to assess myocardial damage in patients with suspected myocarditis and cardiac rejection. J Nucl Med 1988; 29:1893-1900.

15. Obrador D, Ballester M. Carrio I et al. Active myocardial damage with out attending inflammatory response in dilated cardiomyopathy. J Am Coll Cardiol 1993; 14:1667-1671.

16. Khaw BA, Klibanov A, O'Donnel SM et al. Gamma imaging with negatively charge modified monoclonal antibody: modification with synthetic polymers. J Nucl Med 1991; 32:1742-1751.

17. Wiseman J, Rouleau J, Rigo P. Strauss HW, Pitt B. Gallium-67 myocardial imaging for the detection of bacterial endocarditis. Radiology 1976; 120:135-138.

18. Melvin ET, Berger M, Lutzker LG et al. Noninvasive methods for detection of valve vegetations in infective endocarditis. Am J Cardiol 1981: 47;271-278.

19. Morguet AJ, Munz DL, Ivancevic V et al. Immunoscintigraphy using technetium-99m-labelled anti-NCA-95 antigranulocyte antibodies as an adjunct to echocardiography in subacute infective endocarditis. J Am Cardiol 1994; 23:1171-1178.

20. Bourke SJ, Banham SW, McKillop JH, Boyd G. Clearance of 99mTc-DTPA in pigeon fancier's hypersensitivity pneumonitis. Am Rev Respir Dis 1990; 142:1168-1171.

21. Rinderknecht J, Shapiro L, Krauthammer M et al. Accelerated clearance of small solvents from the lungs in interstitial lung disease. Am Rev Respir Dis 1980; 121:105-117.

22. Susskind H, Weber DA, Volkow ND et al. Increased lung permeability following longterm use of free-base cocaine (crack) Chest 1991; 100:903-909.

23. Labrune S. Chinet Th, Collignon L, Barritault L, Huchon GJ. Mechanisms of increased epithelial clearance of DTPA in diffuse fibrosing alveolitis. Eur Respir J 1994; 7:651-656.

24. Wells AU, Hansell DM, Harrison NK et al. Clearance of inhaled ^{99m}Tc DTPA predicts the clinical course of fibrosing alveolitis. Eur Respir J 1993; 6:797-802.

25. Uh S, Lee SM, Kim HT, Chung Y, Kim YH, Park CS. The clearance rate of alveolar epithelium using 99mTc-DTPA in patients with diffuse infiltrating lung disease. Chest 1994; 106:161-165.

26. Line BR, Fulmer JD, Reynolds HY et al. Gallium-67 citrate scanning in the staging of idiopathic pulmonary fibrosis: Correlation with physiologic and morphologic faetures and bronchoalveolar lavage. Am Rev Respir Dis 1978; 118:355-365.

27. Line BR, Hunninghake GW, Keogh BA et al. Gallium-67 scanning to stage the alveolitis of sarcoidosis: correlation with clinical studies, pulmonary function studies and bronchoalveolar lavage. Am Rev Respir Dis 1981; 123:440-446.

28. Crystal RG, Gadek JE, Ferrans VJ, Fulmer JD, Line BR, Hunnignhake GW. Interstitial lung disease: Current concepts of pathogenasis, staging and therapy. Am J Med 1981; 70:542-568.

29. Richman SD, Levenson SM, Bunn PA, Flinn GS, Johnston GS, DeVita VT. Gallium-67 accumulation in pulmonary lesions associated with bleomycin toxicity. Cancer 1975; 36:1966-1972.

30. MacMahon H and Bekerman C. Diagnostic significance of gallium uptake in patients with normal chest radiographs. Radiology 1978; 127:189-193.

31. Siemsen JK, Sargent EN, Grebe SF, Winsor Dw, Jacobsen G. Pulmonary concentration of Ga67 in pneumoconiosis. Am J Roentgenol 1974; 120:815-820.

32. Bekerman C, Hoffner PB, Bitran JD, Gupta RG. Gallium-67 citrate imaging studies of the lung. Semin Nucl Med 1980; 10:286-301.

33. Mason GR, Effros RM, Uszler JM et al. Small solute clearance from the lungs of patients with cardiogenic and noncardiogenic pulmonary edema. Chest 1985; 88:327-334.

34. Terra-Filho M. Vargas FS, Meneguetti JC et al. Pulmonary clearance of technetium 99m diethylene triamine penta acetic acid aerosol in patients with amiodarone pneumonitis. Eur J Nucl Med 1990; 17:334-337.

35. O'Doherty MJ, Van de Pette JEW, Page CJ, Bateman NT, Singh AK, Croft DN. Pulmonary permeability in haematological malignancies: Effects of the disease and cytotoxic agents. Cancer 1986; 58:1286-1288.

36. Chopra SK, Taplin GV, Tashkin DP, Elam D. Lung clearance of soluble radioaerosols of different molecular weights in systemic sclerosis. Thorax 1979; 34:63-67.

37. Niden AH and Mishkin FS. Clinical usefulness of gallium lung scans. Compr Ther 1979; 5:24-34.

38. Basran GS, Byrne AJ, Hardy JG. A noninvasive technique for monitoring lung vascular permeability in man. Nucl Med Commun 1985; 3:3-10.

39. Braude S, Apperley J, Krausz T, Goldman JM, Royston D. Adult respiratory distress syndrome after allogeneic bone marrow transplantation: Evidence for a neutrophil independent mechanism. Lancet 1985; 1:1239-1242.

40. Kaplan JD, Calandrino FS, Schuster DP. A positron emission tomographic comparison of pulmonary vascular permeability during the adult respiratory distress syndrome and pneumonia. Am Rev Respir Dis 1991; 143:150-154.

41. Velazquez M, Weibel ER, Kuhn C et al. PET evaluation of pulmonary vascular permeability: a structure-function-correlation. J Appl Physiol 1991; 70:2206-2216.

42. Mintun MA, Dennis DR, Welch MJ, Mathias CJ, Schuster DP. Measurements of pulmonary vascular permeability with PET and gallium-68-transferrin. J Nucl Med 1987; 28:1704-1716.

43. Mintum MA, Warfel TE, Schuster DP. Evaluating pulmonary vascular permeability with radiolabelled proteins: an error analysis. J Appl Physiol 1990; 68:1696-1706.

44. Jefferies AL, Coates G, O'Brodovich H. Pulmonary epithelial permeability in hyaline membrane disease. N Eng J Med 1984; 131:1075-1080.
45. Sulavik SB, Spencer RP, Palestro CJ et al. Specificity and sensitivity of distinctive chest radiographic and/or 67Ga images in the noninvasive diagnosis of sarcoidosis. Chest 1993; 103:403-409.
46. Sulavik SB, Spencer RP, Weed DA, Shapiro HR, Shiue S, Castriotta RJ. Recognition of distinctive patterns of gallium-67 distribution in sarcoidosis. J Nucl Med 1990; 31:1909-1914.
47. Baughman RP, Fernandez M, Bosken C. Comparison of gallium-67 scanning, bronchoalveolar lavage and serum angiotensin-convering enzymelevels in pulmonary sarcoidosis: predicting response to therapy. Am Rev Respir Dis 1984; 129:676.
48. Lawrence EC, Teague RB, Gottlieb MS. Serial changes in markers of disease activity with corticosteroid treatment in sarcoidosis. Am J Med 1983; 74:747.
49. Alberts C, Van der Schoot JB. Standardized quantitative 67Ga scintigraphy in pulmonary sarcoidosis. Sarcoidosis 1988; 5:111-118.
50. Lewis PJ. Salama A. Uptake of fluorine-18-fluorodeoxyglucose in sarcoidosis. J Nucl Med 1994; 35:1647-1649.
51. Valind SO, Rhodes CG, Paltin C, Suzuki T, Hughes JMB. Measurements of pulmonary glucose metabolism in patients with cryptogenic fibrosing alveolitis and pulmonary sarcoidosis. Am Rev Respir Dis 1984; 129:A53.
52. Brudin LH, Valind SO, Rhodes CG et al. Fluorine-18 deoxyglucose uptake in sarcoidosis measured with positron emission tomography. Eur J Nucl Med 1994; 21:297-305.
53. Kubota R, Yamada S, Kubota K, Ishiwata K, Tamahashi N, Ido T. Intratumoral distribution of fluoride-18-fluorodeoxyglucose in vivo: high accumulation in macrophages and granulocytes studied by microautoradiography. J Nucl Med 1992; 33:1972-1980.
54. Chinet T, Jaubert F, Dusser D, Danel C, Chretien J, Huchon GJ. Effects of inflammation and fibrosis on pulmonary function in diffuse lung fibrosis. Thorax 1990; 45:675-678.
55. Dusser DJ, Collignon MA, Stanislas-Leguern G, Barritault LG, Chretien J, Huchon GJ. Respiratory clearance of 99mTc DTPA and pulmonary involvement in sarcoidosis. Am Rev Respir Dis 1986; 134:493-497.
56. Watanabe N, Inoue T, Oriuchi H, Suzuki H, Hirano T, Endo K. Increased pulmonary clearance in aerosolised 99Tcm-DTPA in patients with a subset of stage I sarcoidosis. Nucl Med Commun 1995; 16: 464-467.
57. Vanhagen PM, Krenning EP, Reubi JC et al. Somatostatin analogue scintigraphy in granulomatous disease. Eur J Nucl Med 1994; 21:497-502.
58. Diot R, Lemarie E, Baulie JL et al. Scintigraphy with J001 macrophage targeting glycolipeptide. A new approach for sardoisosis imaging. Chest 1992; 102:670-676.
59. Jonker ND, Peters AM, Gaskin G, Pusey CD, Lavender JP. A retrospective study of radiolabeled granulocyte kinetics in patients with systemic vasculitis. J Nucl Med 1992; 33:491-497.
60. Wraight EP, Llewellyn MB, Lockwood CM. Indium-111 leucocyte imaging in systemic vasculitis. Nucl Med Commun 1990; 11:201-202.
61. Thadepalli H, Rambhatla K, Mishkin FS, Khurana M, Niden AH. Correlation of microbiologic findings and [67]gallium scans in patients with pulmonary infections. Chest 1977; 72:442-448.
62. Patz EF, Lowe VJ, Hoffman JM et al. Focal pulmonary abnormalities: evaluation with F-18 fluorodeoxyglucose PET scanning. Radiology 1993; 188:487-490.
63. Currie DC, Saverymuttu SH, Peters AM et al. Indium-111 labelled granulocyte accumulation in the respiratory tract of patients with bronchiectasis. Lancet 1987; 1:1335-1339.
64. Saverymuttu SH, Phillips G, Peters AM, Lavender JP. III-Indium autologous leucocyte scanning in lobar pneumonia and lung abscesses. Thorax 1985; 40:925-930.
65. Murray JF, Garay SM, Hopewell PC, Mills J, Snider GL, Stover DE. Pulmonary complications of the acquired immunodeficiency syndrome: an update. Am Rev Respir Dis 1987; 135:504-509.

66. O'Doherty MJ, Breen D, Page CJ, Barton I, Nunan TO. Lung 99m-Tc DTPA transfer in renal disease and pulmonary infection. Nephrol Dial Transplant 1991; 6:582-587.

67. Coleman D, Hattner R, Luce J. Dodek P, Golden J, Murray J, Correlation between gallium lung scans and fibreoptic bronchoscopy in patients with suspected pneumocystis carinii pneumonia and the acquired immune deficiency syndrome. Am Rev Respir Dis 1984; 130:1166-1169.

68. Kramer EL, Sanger JJ, Garay SM, Grossman R, Tiu S, Banner H. Diagnostic implications of Ga-67 chest scan patterns in human immunodeficiency virus seropositive patients. Radiology 1989; 170:671-676.

69. Hecht D, Snydman D, Crumpacker C, Werner B, Heinz-Lacey B. Gancyclovir for treatment of renal transplant associated primary cytomegalovirus pneumonia. J Infect Dis 1988; 157:186-189.

70. O'Doherty MJ, Revell P, Page CJ, Lee S, Mountford PJ, Numan TO. Donor leucocyte imaging in patients with AIDS. A preliminary communication. Eur J Nucl Med 1990; 17:327-333.

71. Fineman DS, Palestro CJ, Kim CK et al. Detection of abnormalities in febrile AIDS patients with In-111-labelled leucocyte and Ga-67 scintigraphy. Radiology 1989; 170:677-680.

72. Prvulovich EM, Miller RF, Costa DC et al. Immunoscintigraphy with a ^{99}Tc^M-labelled anti-granulocyte monoclonal antibody in patients with human immunodeficiency virus infection and AIDS. Nucl Med Commun 1995; 16:838-845.

73. Cordes M, Roll D, Langer M, Ruhnke M et al. Diagnostic value of early gallium-67 scans (4 h p.i.) in patients with AIDS and PCP. Eur J Nucl Med 1989; 15:172.

74. Bitran J, Beckerman C, Weinstein R, Bennet C, Ryo U, Pinsky S. Patterns of gallium-67 scintigraphy in patients with acquired syndrome and the AIDS related complex. J Nucl Med 1987; 28:1103-1106.

75. Kramer EL, Sanger JJ, Garay SM et al. Gallium-67 scans of the chest in patients with acquired immunodeficiency syndrome. J Nucl Med 1987; 28:1107-1114.

76. Miller RF. Nuclear medicine and AIDS. Eur J Nucl Med 1990; 16:103-118.

77. Palestro CJ,. The current role of gallium imaging in infection. Seminars in Nucl Med 1994; 24:128-141.

78. Tumeh SS, Belville JS, Pugatch R, McNeil B. Ga-67 scintigraphy and computed tomography in the diagnosis of pneumocystis carinii pneumonia in patients with AIDS. A prospective comparison. Clin Nucl Med 1992; 17:387-394.

79. Tuazon CV, Delaney MD, Simon GL et al. Utility of gallium-67 scintigraphy and bronchial washings in the diagnosis and treatment of pneumocystis carinii pneumonia in patients with the acquired immunodeficiency syndrome. Am Rev Respir Dis 1985; 132:1087-1092.

80. Woolfenden JM, Carrasquillo JA, Larson SM et al. Acquired immunodeficiency syndrome. Ga-67 citrate imaging. Radiology 1987; 162:383-387.

81. Bradburne RM, Ettensohn DB, Opal SM, McCool FD. Relapse pf pneumocystis carinii pneumonia in the upper lobes during aerosol pentamidine prophylaxis. Thorax 1989, 44:591-593.

82. Schiff RG, Kabat L, Kamain N et al. Gallium scanning in lymphoid interstitial pneumonitis in children with AIDS. J Nucl Med 1987; 28:1915-1919.

83. Ognibene FP, Masur H, Rogers P et al. Nonspecific interstitial pneumonitis without evidence of pneumocystis carinii in asymptomatic patients infected with human immunodeficiency virus (HIV). Ann Intern Med 1988; 109:179-183.

84. Fischman JA, Strauss HW, Fischman AJ et al. Imaging of pneumocystis carinii pneumonia with ^{111}In-labelled non-specific polyclonal IgG: an experimental study in rats. Nucl Med Commun 1991; 12:175-187.

85. Rubin RH, Fischman AJ, Gallahan RJ et al. III-In-labelled nonspecific immunoglobulin scanning in the detection of focal infection. N Engl J Med 1989; 321:935-940.

86. Rubin RH, Fischman AJ, Needleman M et al. Radiolabelled, nonspecific, polyclonal human immunoglobulin in the detection of focal inflammation by scintigraphy: comparison with gallium-67 citrate and Technetium-99m-labelled albumin. J Nucl Med 1989; 30:385-389.

87. Buscombe J, Lui D, Ensing G, De Jong R, Ell PJ. ^{99m}Tc human immunoglobulin (HIgG): first results of a new agent for the localisation of infection and inflammation. Eur J Nucl Med 1990; 16:649-655.

88. Buscombe J, Oyen WJG, Grant A et al. Indium-111-labelled polyclonal human immunoglobulin: Identifying focal infection in patients positive for human immunodeficiency virus. J Nucl Med 1993; 34:1621-1625.

89. Goldenberg DM, Sharkey RM, Udem S et al. Immunoscintigraphy of pneumocystis carinii pneumonia in AIDS patients. J Nucl Med 1994; 35:1028-1034.

90. Rosso J, Guillon JM, Parrot A et al. Technetium-99m-DTPA aerosol and gallium-67 scanning in pulmonary complications of human immunodeficiency virus infection. J Nucl Med 1992; 33:81-87.

91. O'Doherty MJ, Page CJ, Bradbeer CS et al. The place of lung ^{99m}Tc-DTPA aerosol transfer in the investigation of lung infections in HIV positive patients. Resp Med 1989; 83:395-401.

92. Leach R, Davidson C, O'Doherty MJ, Nayagam M, Tang A, Bateman N. Noninvasive management of fever and breathlessness in HIV positive patients. Eur J Resp Med 1991; 4:19-25.

93. Van der Wall H, Murray IPC, Jones PD, Mackey DWJ, Walker BM, Monaghan P. Optimising technetium 99m diethylene triamine penta-acetate lung clearance in patients with the acquired immunodeficiency syndrome. Eur J Nucl Med 1991; 18:235-240.

94. Robinson DS, Cunningham DA, Dave S, Fleming J, Mitchell DM. Diagnostic value of lung clearance of 99mTc DTPA compared with other non-invasive investigations in pneumocystis carinii pneumonia in AIDS. Thorax 1991; 46:722-726.

95. O'Doherty MJ. ^{99m}Tc DTPA transfer/permeability in patients with HIV disease. J Nucl Med 1995; 39:231-242.

96. Monaghan P, Provan I, Murray C et al. An improved radionuclide technique for the detection of altered pulmonary permeability. J Nucl Med 1991; 32:1945-1949.

97. O'Doherty MJ, Barrington SF, Campbell M, Lowe J, Bradbeer CS. PET scanning in patients with HIV disease. Eur J Nucl Med 1995; 5: 918 (Abstract).

98. Lisbona R, Hakim TS, Dean GW et al. Regional pulmonary perfusion following heart lung transplantation. J Nucl Med 1989; 30:1297-1301.

99. Skeens JL, Fuhrman CR, Yousem SA. Bronchiolitis obliterans in heart-lung transplantation patients. AJR 1989; 153:253-256.

100. Herve PA, Silbert D, Mensch J et al. Increased lung clearance of 99mTc DTPA in allograft lung rejection. The Paris-Sud Lung Transplant Group. Am Rev Respir Dis 1991; 144:1333-1336.

CHAPTER 6

PYREXIA OF UNKNOWN ORIGIN

A. M. Peters and D. Shnier

Introduction

In the last 15 years, the indications for inflammation imaging have changed, largely for two
reasons; firstly, the number of patients with an increased predisposition to infection,
especially immunocompromised patients, has increased, and secondly, developments in
interventional radiology have led to an increasing number of soft tissue abscesses being
diagnosed and drained by radiologists without referral for a leucocyte scan. The challenge
to nuclear medicine, therefore, is now the localisation of pathology in patients referred
with fever but no diagnosis, a clinical presentation called, often imprecisely, pyrexia of
unknown origin (PUO).

Undiagnosed fever can be subdivided into PUO and occult infection.

PUO. Strictly speaking this should be reserved for a subgroup who meet the criteria of
PUO as defined by Larson et al [1] of fever of at least 3 weeks duration, including one
week of in-hospital investigation, with no clue as to the cause.

Occult infection. Patients who are suspected of harbouring infection and who present with
a fever but no definite localising clues. Unlike PUO, patients with occult infection often
have a significant previous medical history, such as diabetes mellitus or recent surgery, but,
as in PUO, data localising the pathology are missing.

Probably the majority of patients labelled as PUO fall into this category.

Only a few papers have been dedicated to the problem of PUO, and most cases of PUO
reported in the literature have been included as small subgroups of larger, more diverse
patient populations. Several problems emerge when reviewing this literature. a) A final
diagnosis is not available in a large proportion of the patients. b) There is often difficulty
obtaining proof that a scintigraphic abnormality is in fact the cause of the fever. c) The
value of a true negative is questionable since in the clinical setting of PUO, negatives (true

P. H.Cox and J. R. Buscombe (eds.), The Imaging of Infection and Inflammation, 117–139.
© 1998 *Kluwer Academic Publishers. Printed in the Netherlands.*

or false) are not generally helpful. d) Strict criteria for PUO are seldom adhered to. In this respect, several end-points have been used in the evaluation of agents for the assessment of undiagnosed fever, including, in decreasing order of specificity, pyogenic infection, any infection, any inflammation, the pathology responsible for the fever and any pathology. Using the last mentioned, specificity by definition would be 100%.

Scintigraphic approach tothepatient with an undiagnosed fever.

The most widely used agents for the detection of pathology in undiagnosed fever are Ga-67, leucocytes labelled with Tc-99m or In-111, and polyclonal human immunoglobulin (HIG), usually labelled with In-111. The normal distribution of Ga-67 includes the reticuloendothelial system, breasts, gut and genitalia (Fig. 1). HIG has a normal distribution which is essentially confined to the blood pool.

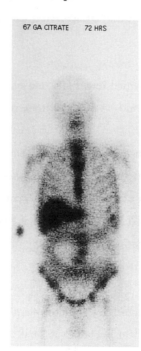

Figure 1. *Ga anterior whole body scan 72 hours post injection. Normal Gallium scan. Note the normal bowel and liver activity. There is prominent bone barrow uptake as a result of chronic stimulation.*

Labelled leucocytes have a rather complex normal distribution based on physiological neutrophil pooling which occurs predominantly in the reticuloendothelial system and to a lesser extent the lung.

Ga-67

The purpose of the Ga-67 scan is not primarily to make a diagnosis, but to localise a potential cause which can then be further investigated with other modalities, such as ultrasound, CT or MRI. Clinical accuracy figures for Ga-67 should therefore be based on an end-point of localisation of any pathology rather than on its ability to identify infection/inflammation. Ga-67 is the agent of choice in (true) PUO and arguably in cases of occult infection of greater than 2 weeks duration.

Ga-67 is taken up into abnormal tissue by several mechanisms, including increased vascular permeability to the Ga-67 transferrin complex formed in vivo following intravenous injection of Ga-67-citrate.

Increased Ga-67 uptake may be seen with:

* Infections, both pyogenic abscesses, and non pyogenic infection such as tuberculosis.
* Tumours, particularly lymphoma and melanoma.
* Inflammatory conditions such as sarcoidosis and vasculitis (Fig. 2 & 3).

Abdominal abscesses, and particularly inflammatory bowel disease (IBD), as causes of PUO may be difficult to diagnose with Ga-67 because of the non-specific bowel activity. Repeat views the next day may help. Patients with haematological conditions often show a strikingly abnormal biodistribution of Ga-67. Uniform increased uptake may be seen in an expanded red marrow (Fig. 1). Free Ga-67 is a bone-seeking radiopharmaceutical and skeletal uptake reflecting increased bone turnover may be seen, as, for example, in degenerative joint disease. When given to patients who have received several blood transfusions or who have saturated their transferrin binding sites for other reasons, Ga-67 may give rise to a skeletal image resembling a bone scan, combined with prominent urinary and parenchymal renal activity. Active bone marrow uptake, in contrast, is of the gallium-transferrin complex.

Ga-67 is often useful in undiagnosed fever, especially PUO. Its value for imaging inflammation was first reported by Lavender and his colleagues [2].

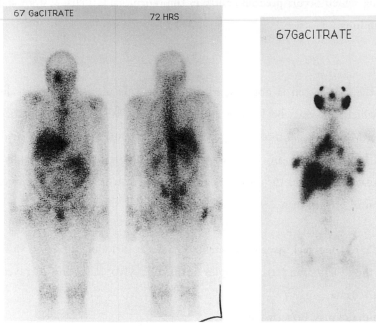

Fig.2   Fig.3

Figure 2. *Ga anterior and posterior whole body scan 72 hours post injection.   Wegener's granulomatosis.   Increase in renal and nasal uptakecan be seen.   This is typical of this condition. The shoulder uptake is related to arthritis.   Prominent uptake adjacent to the rigb hip is due to inflammation at the site of intramuscular injection.   Note the normal bowel and liver activity.*

Figure 3. *Ga anterior whole body scan 72 hours post injection.   Sarcoidosis.   The prominent parotid, lacrimal, hilar and mediastinal uptake that can be seen are typical of this disease.   The axillary and splenic uptake are unusual.   The differential includes lymphoma, TB and complications of HIV.   This illustrates the sensitive but non specific nature of Gallium.*

Early studies, often loosely defined, confirmed the value of Ga-67 in PUO [3,4]. In the study by Sfakianakis et al [4] of 32 patients with undiagnosed fever, 26 had sites of proven infection. All 7 false negative In-111-leucocyte scans were obtained in patients whose fever exceeded two weeks, whilst all 5 false negative Ga-67 scans occurred in patients with fever of less than one week. They concluded that for occult fever of more than two weeks, Ga-67 is indicated.

Leucocyte scintigraphy

The purpose of the leucocyte scan is to identify areas of occult infection and allow their further evaluation, and possibly treatment, by other imaging modalities. Hence the pretest distinction between PUO and occult infection is important. The likelihood of a positive leucocyte scan is higher if clinical circumstances indicate the fever is due to a pyogenic organism, particularly if a bacteraemia is present. Indicators of occult infection include bacteraemia, a history of recent surgery and other high risk factors such as diabetes or immunosuppression.

In-111 leucocytes have a theoretical advantage over Tc-99m in chronic infection that has not been convincingly borne out in limited studies.

Labelled neutrophils have a relatively short residence time in the circulation (about 10 hr) before they are removed by the reticuloendothelial system [5]. They accumulate at sites of inflammation through binding to endothelial adhesion molecules [6]. It can be appreciated from table 1 that most causes of PUO are not associated with a neutrophilic infiltrate. Successful imaging with radiolabelled leucocytes requires an inflammatory process predominantly involving neutrophils. Most causes of PUO have a predominantly monocytic and/or lymphocytic infiltrate and are unlikely to give a positive leucocyte scan. Claims that the lymphocytic contamination of a mixed cell population is responsible for visualization of some chronic infections (thereby implying a superior performance for mixed cells in comparison with pure granulocytes) are not supported by experimental data which show that lymphocytes are highly radio-sensitive and would not survive after exposure to the levels of In-111 encountered in routine mixed leucocyte labelling [7]. In contrast to PUO, occult infection is more likely to be associated with a neutrophilic infiltrate. Because the infection is likely to have become prolonged, by the time the patient is referred for a nuclear medicine study it may have become associated with a mixed or predominantly monocytic infiltrate.

Distinguishing between PUO and occult infection is useful for two reasons: firstly and most importantly, it helps choose between a leucocyte scan or a less specific alternative, such as Ga-67; and secondly it helps to classify and interpret the nuclear medicine literature in this area, which has focused predominantly on occult infection while claiming to address PUO. Because of several factors pointing to pyogenic infection, patients classified as having occult infection are more usefully investigated with labelled leucocytes, whereas patients with PUO should probably be investigated with a less specific tracer, such as Ga-67. When using labelled leucocytes to investigate undiagnosed fever, there is a choice between In-111-labelled mixed leucocytes, In-111-labelled pure granulocytes, Tc-99m-labelled leucocytes. Radiolabelled lymphocytes are highly radiosensitive, and are of no value for the assessment of undiagnosed fever. There is very little data in the literature on which to guide a choice between the other preparations.

It will depend to some extent on local conditions and theoretical considerations. Thus, although pure neutrophils might be expected to perform better than mixed leucocytes in PUO, because a greater fraction of the injected label is associated with migrating cells, the literature suggests that they perform equally well [8].

Two papers, both based on small numbers, have examined the value of In-111-leucocytes in PUO [9,10]. In both studies, there was a high proportion of patients in whom no final diagnosis was reached and neither was able to demonstrate any correlation between leucocytosis and image positivity. The leucocyte scan was, however, more frequently positive in patients with a history of surgery within 6 months. A valuable study by Syrjala et al [11] defined the value of In-111-leucocytes in patients with fever of two or more weeks, who they divided into three groups: socalled PUO (ie, no clues present); post operative; and those with bacteraemia of at least one week. The end point of the study was infection. The yield of true positives (28%) was the same in post-operative patients as in PUO, but bacteraemia gave a significantly higher yield (68%). Although a correlation was seen between a positive result and a raised CRP, it was based on all three groups. Whereas the authors therefore concluded that CRP was a useful guideline, this may not have necessarily been the case in the difficult PUO group alone.

On theoretical grounds, Tc-99m-leucocytes should be less useful than In-111-leucocytes because although they provide better photon flux and image resolution, infections in undiagnosed fever are usually chronic, low grade or induce a mononuclear infiltrate, all of which result in a critical dependence on 24 hours imaging. Tc-99m is less stable in both labelled cells and targeted inflammatory tissue [12]; along with a shorter physical half-life and non-specific bowel activity, this reduces the reliability of 24 hour imaging. A poor performance in comparison with In-111 has not, however, been demonstrated. Few studies in PUO have been carried out with Tc-99m labelled cells [13-15]. It is of interest that in two studies of Tc-99m-HMPAO-leucocytes from Vorne's group, one in comparison with Ga-67 [13] and the other with Tc-99m HIG [14], there were 9 patients with PUO, 8 of whom were classified as true negative and one as true positive. Of 5 that received Ga-67, 4 were classified as true negative and one, with a malignancy, classified as false negative (which was true positive on the Tc-99m white cell scan). The 3 true negatives all had malignancies and so may well have been positive with Ga-67. This study illustrates the need to carefully define what constitutes a true positive (perhaps better described as "useful" positive) in this particular clinical setting.

Radiolabelled human immunoglobulin (HIG)

When HIG was introduced as an inflammation imaging agent [16], hopes were raised that it would be specific and sensitive for infection on the basis of binding of the Fc portion of the IgC molecule to local Fc receptors at sites of inflammation [17]. Although this turned out not to be the case, interest in HIG was maintained by the publication of several articles showing an accuracy which matched In-111-leucocyte scanning [18,19]. HIG is a rational alternative to Ga-67 for investigating undiagnosed fever since it is a marker of increased endothelial permeability and, like the gallium-transferrin complex, accumulates at sites of pathology as a result of non-specific "leakage" into the interstitial space across a compromised endothelium [20]. Having entered the interstitial space, In-111 transchelates from HIG to local protein, including lactoferrin, leaving the intact HIG to diffuse back into plasma [21]. This results in progressive accumulation of label at the inflammatory site. Images become increasingly positive over several days after injection of the agent. A similar mechanism probably occurs with Ga-67, which becomes bound extravascularly by host and bacterial protein (lactoferrin and siderophores, respectively). Tc-99m-HIG, on the other hand, appears to be stable extravascularly, with no translocation of label. This represents a significant disadvantage of Tc-99m HIG. Most publications have compared In-11-HIG with labelled leucocytes, but, because of its kinetics of uptake, a more rational comparison would perhaps be with Ga-67.

Regional pathology as a cause of undiagnosed fever.
Soft tissue sepsis

Soft tissue sepsis in a limb is usually evident on clinical examination; it may produce strikingly abnormal uptake on a white cell scan (Fig. 4). There is often a history of previous trauma, or an abscess may develop at the site of frequent previous intramuscular injections. Soft tissue sepsis evident on a white cell scan may nevertheless not be the cause of the patient's fever and it is important to search elsewhere with whole body scanning.

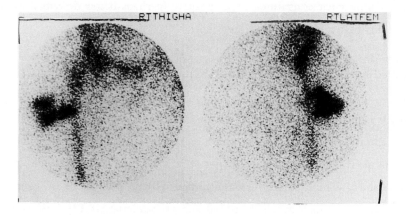

Figure 4. *In-111 Leukocyte scan 24 hours post injection, AP and lateral right thigh. A large soft tissue abscess in a patient presenting with bacteraememia and positive blood cultures. Note the normal bone marrow uptake.*

Intrathoracic disease

Intrathoracic diseases which may present as an undiagnosed fever include pyogenic processes, such as bronchiectasis, malignancies, particularly lymphoma, infectious and non infectious granulomatous disease, including tuberculosis and sarcoidosis, and pulmonary vasculitis.

Although usually used for the follow-up of disease activity in sarcoidosis, Ga-67 imaging may help to suggest this diagnosis in a patient presenting with PUO. Ga-67 can be very helpful, not by establishing the cause of the PUO, but by localising pathology and directing further imaging such as computerised tomography (CT). Abnormal uptake of Ga-67 at extra-thoracic sites of sarcoidosis (excluding salivary and lacrimal gland uptake) is unusual (Fig.3). With Ga-67, intrathoracic tuberculosis gives similar appearances to sarcoidosis. Abnormal parotid gland uptake is not specific for sarcoidosis. It may bee seen in a variety of illnesses, including tuberculosis and in any debilitated patient with chronic low grade sialadenitis. Extra-thoracic abnormalities are more common in tuberculosis.

Various approaches for quantifying Ga-67 uptake in sarcoidosis, which may be useful for assessing disease activity, have been proposed but are not widely used. In general, they derive ratios of counts per pixel at abnormal sites in comparison with reference regions such as liver, bone marrow or irrelevant soft tissue. Ga-67 is also taken up by several pulmonary neoplasms, especially lung cancer, but has no clearly established role in their management. It is, however, useful in a variety of other inflammatory diseases of the lung, such as fungal infections, and in particular opportunist infections in immuno-compromised patients, such as PCP. For the latter, it is being increasingly used in the management of HIV-positive patients [22].

On leucocyte scintigraphy bronchiectasis shows as focal, often multiple, accumulations usually with a bronchopulmonary segmental or lobar distribution [23]. (Fig. 5).

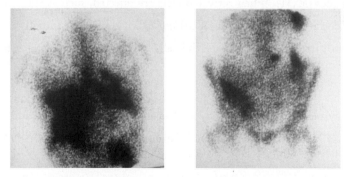

Figure 5. *In-111 leucocyte scan 24 hours post injection, anterior chest and abdomen. Bronchiectasis with widespread abnormal neutrophil accumulation in the right lower lobe. Extensive bowel activity is due to swallowed granulocytes. The bowel was normal on the 3 hour image (not shown)*

There is usually evidence of enteric In-111 activity as a result of swallowed labelled sputum. Currie et al [23] observed that about one third of bronchiectatic lobes were negative on leucocyte scanning and positive on CT, but the reverse was rarely seen. These were not false negatives but instead indicated quiescent disease in the presence of a structural abnormality. In contract to bronchiectasis, lobar pneumonia is usually negative on leucocyte scintigraphy [24]. In experimental streptococcal lobar pneumonia, Clark et al [25] demonstrated that In-111 labelled granulocyte migration into the involved lobe terminated within 24 hr of lobar instillation of the bacteria but increased F-18 labelled deoxyfluoroglucose (FDG) uptake, reflecting the granulocyte respiratory burst, commenced later and persisted for longer. This has since been demonstrated in human pneumonia [26]. In bronchiectasis, however, whereas leucocyte scintigraphy is frequently dramatically positive, FDG scans have been unimpressive, which along with the data from pneumonia, underlines the dissociation between neutrophil migration and subsequent neutrophil metabolic activity [26].

The physiology of granulocyte traffic through the lung is controversial. Some authors consider the pulmonary vascular bed to be the major site in the body for granulocyte margination whilst others think that it represents no more than the average for the whole body [27,28,29]. Early prominent lung activity is well-recognised following the injection of labelled granulocytes for clinical use, and the intensity has been shown to correlate with labelling techniques [30,31]. When activated cells are injected, such as following isolation on saline-based density gradient columns, the lung activity, although initially marked, clears quite rapidly with irreversible uptake of the cells by the liver and, to a lesser extent, the spleen [30].

Patients with systemic vasculitis, such as Wegener's granulomatosis and microscopic polyarteritis, may be referred for leucocyte scanning for the investigation of undiagnosed fever.

Early images over the lungs show diffusely increased activity which is the result of a genuine, pathophysiologically increased granulocyte margination (i.e. intravascular delay) in the pulmonary vascular bed [32]. Since the delayed cells do not migrate into the pulmonary extravascular space to any significant extent, the lung activity clears over 24 hr, much more slowly than the artefactual lung activity resulting from in vitro cell activation. This slow time course of clearance is consistent with the notion that the early signal in vasculitis arises from granulocytes in dynamic equilibrium between a circulating and pulmonary marginating pool. In contrast to the kinetics associated with in vitro granulocyte activation, there is less liver uptake, and the distribution of granulocytes between liver and spleen remains normal. Other febrile diseases showing a similar, non-artefactual increase in diffuse pulmonary activity include graft versus host disease (Fig. 6) [33], IBD [34], adult respiratory distress syndrome (ARDS) [35] and drug-induced pneumonitis [36].

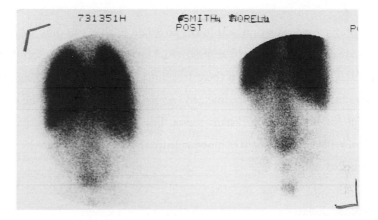

Patients with systemic vasculitis frequently have other manifestations of vasculitis, including renal and gut vasculitis [32]. Wegener's granulomatosis is associated with increased nasal uptake. These patients are occasionally referred for white cell scans because of occult fever, with no suspicion of systemic vasculitis, and the finding of the characteristic lung activity should prompt a search for these other features of vasculitis.

Cardiovascular causes of fever are difficult to image with radionuclides. Leucocyte scintigraphy for endocarditis and valvular vegetations are occasionally requested, but are almost always negative.

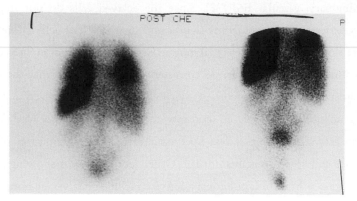

Figure 6 *Tc99m-Leukocyte scan 1 hour (a) and 3 hours (b) post injection, posterior chest and abdomen. Abdominal abscess in a patient with graft versus host disease (GVHD) post bone marrow transplant. Marked diffuse lung uptake is seen, this is often associated with GVHD. The focus of abnormal uptake in the abdomen is due to an abdominal abscess.*

Notwithstanding passive adhesion within the circulation, they can only be positive if the labelled cells are able to migrate into an interstitial location. Leucocyte scans are therefore seldom helpful. On the other hand, if there are clinical reasons for suspecting septic emboli or metastatic abscess arising from the infected vegetations (or vice versa), the white cell scan may be useful for documenting distant sepsis. For the same reason, a patient with an undiagnosed fever who has a positive blood culture should be investigated with leucocytes preferably labelled with In-111.

Intra-abdominal disease

Febrile patients presenting with PUO may harbour intra-abdominal sepsis (Fig.7). This may be subphrenic, intra-hepatic, rarely intra-splenic, perirenal, or exist as free septic fluid in the peritoneal cavity. In many patients a diagnosis is established on ultrasound and/or CT, but when these are negative or are not specific for sepsis, a leucocyte scan is the next option. The approaches to intra-hepatic and sub-phrenic sepsis are rather similar and based on identification of normal liver or splenic tissue. The time course of uptake of cells into the liver and spleen are different from each other and both are different from the time course of uptake into sepsis.

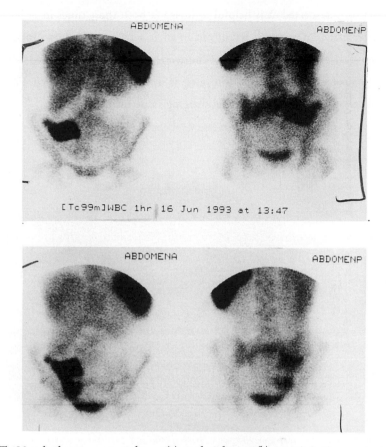

Figure 7. *Tc-99m leukocyte scan 1 hour (a) and 4 hours (b) post injection, anterior and posterior abdomen. Right Iliac fossa abscess secondary to Crohn's disease probably communicating with bowel. Prominent activity in the right iliac fossa presents at one hour (a) is appreciably more extensive at 4 hours (b), suggesting communication of the abscess with the bowel lumen. This patient presented with fever of unknown origin.*

Granulocytes undergo pooling in the spleen and the time course of uptake reflects equilibration of the cells between the pool and circulating blood [37]. Liver uptake reflects several processes including pooling and reversible sequestration, which seems to be related to the degree of cell activation or damage sustained in vitro during labelling. Consequently liver activity is usually more prominent one hour after injection than at 3 hr and, if intra-hepatic sepsis is suspected, it is helpful to image at both these times in order to define the normal liver tissue. In contrast, activity in an enclosed abscess increases progressively with a time-course that is the mirror image of the decreasing circulating labelled cell activity (Fig. 8). Complementary Tc-99m colloid imaging is not usually necessary to make a diagnosis of liver abscess, especially if sequential imaging is performed.

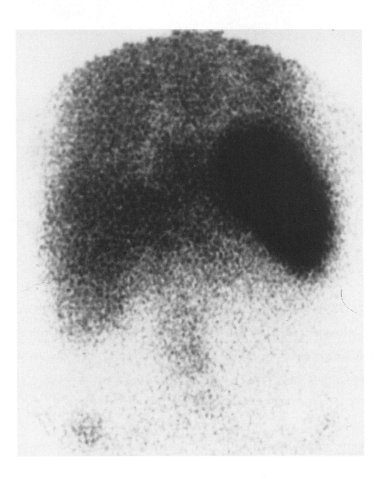

Sequential imaging of suspected abdominal sepsis is particularly important in order to diagnose an abscess in communication with bowel lumen. These are not uncommon and, because of a delay in diagnosis, have a worse prognosis than non-communicating abscess [38]. Ultrasound and CT often miss these lesions because of their spontaneous decompression.

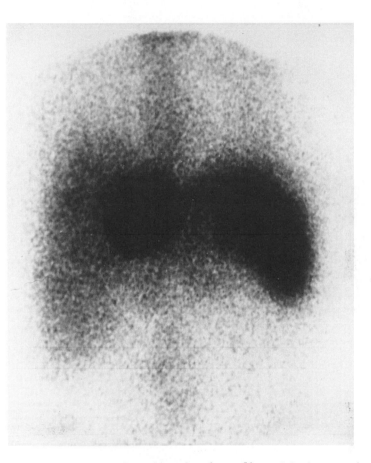

Figure 8. *In-111 leucocyte scan 1 hour (a) and 24 hours (b) post injection, anterior abdomen. Liver abscess. Note the slightly diminished activity in the left lobe of the liver in the 1 hour image with marked increase in focal activity by 24 hours.*

Characteristically, on early imaging, localisation of cells can be seen in the abscess, and this is followed later by evidence of activity in gut lumen (Fig. 9). Because of non-specific bowel activity, a communicating abscess is more difficult to diagnose with Tc-99m than with In-111 labelled cells. Nevertheless, by imaging at one and 3 hr, the change in position of the abnormal activity can be appreciated with Tc-99m and the diagnosis can be made. More slowly decompressing collections are likely to be missed with Tc-99m labelled cells.

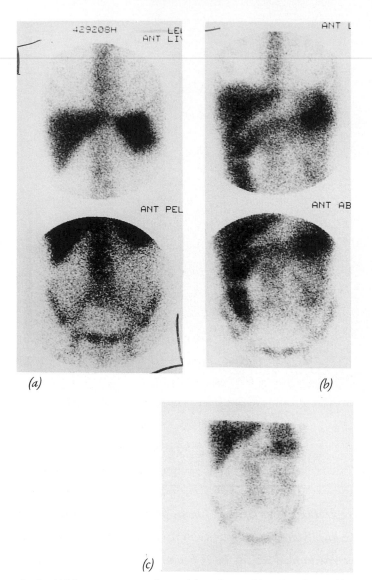

Figure 9. *In-111 leucocyte scan 4 hours (a), 26 hours (b) and 90 hours (c) post injection, anterior abdomen. Splenic flexure abscess communicating with bowel. In retrospect the spleen in (a) is abnormally shaped due to the close proximity of the abscess. Colonic activity present at 26 hours (b) is presumably due to communication with the bowel plus retrograde passage of granulocytes within the colon. (c) demonstrates the residual activity in the abscess more convincingly.*

Swallowed labelled granulocytes from any form of septic lung disease, including chronic bronchitis, can cause a confusing abdominal image 24 hr after labelled granulocyte injection. Failure to perform an image at 3 hr may result in misinterpretation of bowel activity as IBD or abdominal sepsis (Fig.5). With In-111 or Tc-99m labelled granulocytes, IBD and abdominal abscesses are almost always positive by 3 hr.

Postoperative fever

MacSweeney et al [9] observed that the likelihood of PUO being caused by a pyogenic infection was only about 10%, unless the patient had undergone surgery within 6 months of the fever, when the percentage rose to about 50%. Six months is therefore a convenient time after surgery up to which a fever could be described as post-operative. Most post-operative fevers originate within the abdomen. The imaging approach is relatively straightforward and after negative preliminary investigations such as abdominal x-ray and ultrasound, and possibly CT, a white cell scan is the preferred next option.

Tc-99m or In-111 labelled cells can be used, although In-111 may be preferable in view of the possibility of complications such as communication of an intra-abdominal abscess with gut lumen (Fig. 9) or with a hollow viscus, eg rectal or vaginal fistulae. Post-operative patients frequently have draining tubes, so it is helpful to know the surgical procedures that have been undertaken and the sites at which draining tubes have been inserted. It is essential to image the bags into which the tubes drain, otherwise the extent of sepsis may be underestimated, and also to avoid confusion with the normal physiology of the tracer. For instance, tubes draining the hepatobiliary tree will contain Tc-99m labelled secondary HMPAO species, which otherwise give rise to non-specific bowel activity. Because of this handling of Tc-99m it is advisable to use In-111 labelled cells to investigate fevers following hepatobiliary surgery. Changing the patient's position between erect and supine may be helpful, if the patient's condition permits, so as to distinguish between free septic fluid in the abdomen and loculated or enclosed abscesses. If an abdominal abscess is suspected on the basis of a leucocyte scan (Fig. 7), the patient should go immediately to ultrasound or CT even if this was previously unrewarding.

Renal disease

Many patients from the renal unit are referred for leukocyte scintigraphy. They are in general a rather unrewarding group in so far as many have negative studies. Most have chronic renal failure and are being treated with peritoneal or haemodialysis when they present with occult fever. Many have non-functioning allografts in situ. Often, it is uncertain whether fever is due to infected current or old access grafts, infection of a Tenchkoff catheter tunnel or due to an unrelated new focus of sepsis. As for patients with suspected hepatobiliary sepsis, renal patients should in general be investigated with In-111 rather than Tc-99m labelled cells in view of potential confusion caused by renal uptake of secondary HMPAO complexes, which results in parenchymal and urinary activity [39]. A rare but striking finding seen unequivocally only with In-111 is generalised diffuse and symmetrical uptake of leukocytes in the kidneys. This is a feature of vasculitis and in Wegener's granulomatosis, may be associated with increased uptake in the nasal region or with evidence of pulmonary vasculitis (see above). Increased pulmonary activity may also be seen in relation to recent haemodialysis, which causes granulocyte activation [40].

Previously failed transplanted kidneys left in situ may also become infected, although a non-infected, non-functioning allograft may by itself cause fever as a result of immunological intolerance. As most of these patients have occult fever, the decision to perform a Ga-67, HIG or white cell scan may be difficult. Recently, In-111 labelled platelet uptake has been proposed as a means of identifying fever caused by immunological intolerance to a non-functioning graft [41].

Undiagnosed fever in paediatrics

Serious pyogenic infection in an otherwise normal individual seems to be less common in children than in adults. The majority of white cell scans performed in paediatrics are for the investigation of suspected IBD. Others are performed in immunocompromised children or those with inherited diseases such as granulomatous disease, in which the neutrophil is defective in bacterial killing. White cell scanning can be used to localise infections in these children because migration itself is normal. The execution and interpretation of leukocyte scintigraphy in children is in general similar to adults.

Because of a more favourable radiation dose, Tc-99m HMPAO labelled cells are preferred over In-111 labelled cells for children. Nevertheless, because many children referred for white cell scanning have had fever for several days to weeks, and have been extensively investigated by other imaging techniques, In-111 labelled cells still have a role, as in chronic sepsis in general. Leukocyte scintigraphy in small children presents the technical challenge of isolating sufficient cells for labelling. This should not be a significant problem as volumes of blood and labelling reagents can be scaled down, or saline added to the initial blood sample to give a workable volume. It is possible to label cells from as little as 5ml blood.

Conclusion and future projections.

Although leukocyte scintigraphy is the gold standard for imaging inflammation, its main disadvantage is the need for in vitro manipulation of autologous blood. This has provided the impetus to find equally effective which can be given "off-the-self". Because of increased capillary permeability, almost any agent works to some extent and this party explains why so many have been proposed over the last few years. A seminal paper by McAfee et al [42] illustrated the clear superiority of In-111-leukocytes in sepsis compared with several experimental tracers, most of which probably owed their uptake to increased capillary permeability. Monoclonal antibodies against granulocytes have proved useful [43,44] but their availability is limited and, as a more fundamental disadvantage, they predominantly label antigenically positive bone marrow granulocyte precursors, which far outnumber circulating granulocytes. They consequently provide very good images of the bone marrow [45].

In the search for improved specificity in inflammation imaging, labelled antibiotics have been successfully used to image infective as opposed to non-infective inflammation [46]. The clinical circumstances suited to this compound, however, need to be carefully defined because unless a specific diagnostic question is addressed the need for an inflammation scan in a patient with an undiagnosed fever is usually to localise pathology. The presence of bacteraemia, on the other hand, would be a strong indication for an infection-specific agent.

Other novel approaches include radiolabelled chemotactic peptides [47], radiolabelled monoclonal antibodies to endothelium [48], FDG [49] and several large molecules which probably target inflammation non-specifically (eg. biotin-avidin complexes and liposomes). Chemotactic peptides, which are thought to target local activated granulocytes, have been shown to work experimentally but not yet clinically. A variant of this approach is radiolabelled interleukin-2 (IL-2), which targets activated lymphocytes expressing IL-2 receptors [50]. This approach has so far been aimed at a limited number of well-specified chronic diseases associated with a lymphocytic infiltrate but may be useful in undiagnosed fever. In-111-octreotide, which targets somatostatin receptors and is claimed to provide positive images of chronic inflammation, may do so by binding to activated lymphocytes [51].

Imaging inflammation with FDG is based on the principle of an increased metabolic rate of activated inflammatory cells. Tumours also have an increased uptake of FDG but this is not necessarily a disadvantage in undiagnosed fever if the aim of the scan is to localise any pathology, inflammatory or otherwise. A tissue of interest for localising inflammation is the vascular endothelium which becomes activated and expresses antigenic proteins called adhesion molecules on its luminal surface during inflammation [6]. Anti-E-selectin labelled with In-111 has been successfully used for imaging both acute and chronic inflammation [52], and several other adhesion molecules could be targeted using the same principle. One attraction of this approach is accessibility of the antigen to the monoclonal. As an alternative to antibodies, it should be possible to identify, isolate and label surface molecules of leukocytes which are responsible for binding endothelial adhesion molecules, thereby reproducing the effectiveness of white cell scanning.

References

1. Larson EB, Featherstone HJ, Petersdorf RG. Fever of undetermined origin: diagnosis and follow-up of 105 cases, 1970-1980. Medicine 1982;61:269-92.
2. Lavender JP, Lowe J, Barker JR. Ga-67 citrate scanning in neoplastic and inflammatory lesions. Br J Radiol 1971;44:361-6.
3. Hilson AJW, Maisy MN. Gallium-67 scanning in pyrexia of unknown origin. Br J Med 1979;2:1330-1.
4. Sfakianakis GN, Al-Sheikh W, Heal A, et al. Comparison of scintigraphy with ^{111}In leukocytes and ^{67}Ga in the diagnosis of occult sepsis. J Nucl Med 1982;23:618-26.
5. Saverymuttu SH, Peters AM, Keshavarzian A, et al. The kinetics of 111-indium distribution following injection of 111-indium labelled autologous granulocytes in man. Br J Haematol 1985;61:675-85.
6. Chapman PT, Haskard DO, Leukocyte adhesion molecules. Br Med Bull 1995;51:296-311.
7. Chisholm PM, Danpure HJ, Healey G, et al. Cell damage resulting from the labelling of rat lymphocytes and Hela S3 cells with In-111 oxine. J Nucl Med 1979;20:1308-11.
8. Schauwecker DS, Burt RW, Park HM, et al. Comparison of purified indium-111 granulocytes and indium-111 mixed leukocytes for imaging of infections. J Nucl Med 1988;29:23-5.
9. MacSweeney JE, Peters AM, Lavender JP. Indium leucocyte scanning in pyrexia of unknown origin. Clin Radiol 1990;42:414-7.
10. Davies SG, Garvie NW. The role of indium-labelled leucocyte imaging in pyrexia of unknown origin. Br J Radiol 1990;63:850-4.
11. Syrjala MT, Valtonen V, Liewendahl K. Diagnostic significance of indium-111 granulocyte scintigraphy in febrile patients. J Nucl Med 1987;28:155-60.
12. Peters AM, Roddie ME, Danpure HJ, et al. Tc-99m HMPAO labelled leucocytes: comparison with In-111-tropolonate labelled granulocytes. Nucl Med Comm 1988;9:449-63.
13. Vorne M, Soini I, Lantto T, et al. Technetium-99m-HMPAO-labeled leukocytes in detection of inflammatory lesions: comparison with gallium-67 citrate. J Nucl Med 1989;30:1332-6.
14. Hovi I, Taavitsainen M, Lantto T, et al. Technetium-99m-HMPAO-labeled leukocytes and technetium-99m-labeled hyman polyclonal immunoglobulin G in diagnosis of focal purulent disease. J Nucl Med 1993;34:1428-34.
15. Bester MJ, Van Heerden PDR, Klopper JF, et al. Imaging infection and inflammation in an African environment: comparison of [99]Tc[m]-HMPAO-labelled leukocytes and ^{67}Ga-citrate. Nucl Med Comm 1995;16:599-607.
16. Rubin RH, Fischman AJ, Callahan KJ, et al. In-labelled non-specific immunoglobulin scanning in the detection of focal infection. N Engl J Med 1989;321:935-40.
17. Rubin RH, Young LS, Hansen WP, et al. Specific and non-specific imaging of localized Fisher immunotype 1. Pseudomonas aeroginosa infection with radiolabeled monoclonal antibody. J Nucl Med 1988;29:651-6.
18. Oyen WJG, Claessens RAMJ, Van der Meer JWM, et al. Detection of subacute infectious foci with In-111 labelled autologous leukocytes and In-111-labeled human nonspecific immunoglobulin G: a prospective comparative study. J Nucl Med 1991;32:1854-60.
19. Datz FL, Anderson CE, Ahluwalia R, et al. The efficacy of indium-111-polyclonal IgG for the detection of infection and inflammation. J Nucl Med 1994;35:74-83.
20. Rubin RH, Fischman AJ. The use of radiolabeled nonspecific immunoglobulin in the detection of focal inflammation. Semin Nucl Med 1994;24:169-79.
21. Claessens RAMJ, Koenders EB, Boerman OC, et al. Dissociation of indium from indium-111-labelled diethylene triamine penta-acetic acid conjugated non-specific polyclonal human immunoglobulin G in inflammatory foci. Eur J Nucl Med 1995;22:212-9.
22. Palestro CJ. The current role of gallium imaging in infection. Semin Nucl Med 1994;24:128-41.

23. Currie DC, Saverymuttu SH, Peters AM, et al. Indium-111 labelled granulocyte accumulation in the respiratory tract of patients with bronchiectasis. Lancet 1987;1:1335-9.

24. Saverymuttu SH, Philips G. Peters AM, et al. 111-Indium autologous leucocyte scanning in lobar pneumonia and lung abscess. Thorax 1985;40:925-30.

25. Clark RJ, Jones HA, Rhodes CG, et al. Non-invasive assessment in self-limiting pulmonary inflammation by external scintigraphy of 111-In labeled neutrophil influx and by measurement of the local metabolic response with positron emission tomography. Am Rev Resp Dis 1989;139:A58(abstr).

26. Jones HA, Sriskandan S, Peters AM, et al. Metabolic activity of neutrophils is distinct from migration in lobar pneumonia and bronchiectasis. Am J Respir Crit Care Med 1995;151:A343(abstr.).

27. Hogg JC. Neutrophil kinetics and lung injury. Physiol Rev 1987;67:1249-95.

28. MacNee W, Selby C. Nuetrophil kinetics in the lungs. Clin Sci 1990;79:97-107.

29. Peters AM, Allsop P, Stuttle AWJ, et al. Granulocyte margination in the human lung and its response to strenuous exercise. Clin Sci 1992;82:237-44.

30. Saverymuttu SH, Peters AM, Danpure HJ, et al. Lung transit of 111-Indium labelled granulocytes. Relationship to labelling techniques. Scand J Haematol 1983;30:151-60.

31. Haslett C. Guthrie LA, Kopaniak MM, et al. Modulation of the multiple neutrophil functions by preparative methods of trace concentrations of bacterial lipopolysaccaride. Am J Pathol 1985;119:101-10.

32. Jonker N, Peters AM, Gaskin G, et al. A retrospective study of granulocyte kinetics in patients with systemic vasculitis. J Nucl Med 1992;33:491-7.

33. Ussov WY, Peters AM, Glass DM, et al. Measurement of the pulmonary vascular granulocyte pool. J Appl Physiol 1995;78:1388-95.

34. Jonker ND, Peters AM, Carpani de Kaski M, et al. Pulmonary granulocyte margination is increased in patients with inflammatory bowel disease. Nucl Med Comm 1992;13:806-10.

35. Warshawski FJ, Sibald WJ, Driedger AA, et al. Neutrophil-pulmonary interaction in the adult respiratory distress syndrome. Am Rev Respir Dis 1986;133:797-804.

36. Palestro CJ, Padilla ML, Swyer AJ, et al. Diffuse pulmonary uptake of In-111 labelled leukocytes in drug-induced pneumonitis. J Nucl Med 1992;33:1175-7.

37. Peters AM, Saverymuttu SH, Keshavarzian A, et al. Splenic pooling of granulocytes. Cli Sci 1985;68:283-9.

38. Saverymuttu SH, Peters AM, Lavender JP. Clinical importance of enteric communication with abdominal abesses. Br Med J 1985;290:23-7.

39. Roddie ME, Peters AM, Danpure HJ et al. Imaging inflammation with Tc-99m hexamethyl propyleneamineoxime (HMPAO) labelled leucocytes. Radiology 1988;166:767-72.

40. Becker W, Schaefer RM, Borner W. In vivo viability of In-111-labelled granulocytes demonstrated in a sham-dialysis model. Br J Radiol 1989;62:463-7.

41. Torregrosa JV, Bassa P, Lomena FJ, et al. The usefulness of ^{111}In-labeled platelet scintigraphy in the diagnosis of patients with febrile syndrome and non-functioning renal graft. Transplantation 1994;

42. McAfee JG, Gagne G, Subramanian G, et al. The localization of indium-111-leukocytes, gallium-67-polyclonal IgG and other radioactive agents in acute focal inflammatory lesions. J Nucl Med 1991;32:2126-31.

43. Becker W, Goldenberg DM, Wolf F. The use of monoclonal antibodies and antibody fragments in the imaging of infectuous lesions. Semin Nucl Med 1994;24:142-53.

44. Lind P, Langsteger W, Kotringer P, et al. Immunoscintigraphy of inflammatory processes with a technetium-99m-labeled monoclonal antigranulocyte antibody (Mab BW 250/183). J Nucl Med 1990;31:417-23.

45. Reske SN. Marrow scintigraphy. In: Churchill Livingstone, Nuclear medicine in clinical diagnosis and treatment. Murray IPC, Ell PJ, editors, Edinburgh:1994;705-9.

46. Vinjamuri S, Hall AV, Solanki KK, et al. Comparison of ^{99m}Tc-infection with radiolabelled white cell imaging in the evaluation of bacterial infection. Lancet 1996;347:233-5.

47. Fischman AJ, Babich JW, Rubin RH. Infection imaging with technetium-99m-labeled chemotactic peptide analogs. Semin Nucl Med 1994;24:154-68.
48. Jamar F, Chapman PT. Harrison AA, et al. Inflammatory arthritis: imaging of endothelial cell activation with an In-111 labeled F(ab')2 fragment of anti-E-selectin monoclonal antibody. Radiology 1995;194:843-50.
49. Gutowski TD, et al. Experimental studies of ^{18}F-2-fluoro-2-deoxy-D-glucose (FDG) in infections and reactive lymphnodes. J Nucl Med 1992;33:925(abstr.).
50. Chianelli M. Signore A, Biassoni L, et al. In vivo imaging of autoimmunity by 99mTc-interleukin-2. Eur J Nucl Med 1995;22:780(abstr.).
51. Van Hagen PM, Krenning EP, Reubi JC, et al. Somatostatin analogue scintigraphy of malignant lymphomas. Br J Haematol 1993;83:75-9.
52. Chapman PT, Jamar F, Keelan ETM, et al. Imaging endothelial activation in inflammation using a radiolabelled monoclonal antibody against E-selectin. Arthr Rhem (in press).

CHAPTER 7

IMAGING INFECTION IN PATIENTS WITH IMMUNODEFICIENCY AND
MULTI-ORGAN FAILURE

J.R. Buscombe

"Claude (*Bernard*) is right: The organism is nothing, the terrain is everything".
[L.Pasteur ,1895]

The Host

The invasion of the body by micro-organisms results in a complex response from the host.
The simplest components of the response include chemicals such as compliment which act
as a general disinfectant. They are toxic to bacteria, fungi etc. However some bacteria are
able to develop a cell wall which acts as armour and are able to resist such attacks.
Therefore some developed cells such as the natural killer (NK) macrophage will, if
encountering an invading bacterium, phagocytose the invader and attempt to digest it.
Again some bacteria are resistant to this approach and it is unhelpful for viruses. There has
developed a complex system of proteins which are able to identify that an organism is
invading and ensure that it is attacked. These protein consist of two pairs of poly-peptide
chains one shorter than the other. The proteins, immunoglobulin are produced by a
different cell line of T-lymphocytes. Each set of immunoglobulin identify a different
antigen. This antigen is a group of molecules, normally a group of proteins or
carbohydrates on the surface of bacteria, fungi or viruses. When this antigen is presented
then these immunoglobulin, or antibodies, cause stimulation of the particular clone of T-
lymphocytes which will cause an explosive increase in the production of antibodies of
exactly the same pattern to help identify and neutralise similar invading micro-organisms.
These antibodies are able to activate and stimulate other macrophages and these cells via
chemical messages recruit further cells involved in the destruction of invading micro-
organisms to the are of infection. At the site of local infection release of histamine and slow
releasing substance (SRS) results in capillary dilatation and leakage from the capillary wall
of both cellular and the non-cellular elements involved in the bodies response to infection.

141

P. H.Cox and J. R. Buscombe (eds.), The Imaging of Infection and Inflammation, 141–160.
© 1998 Kluwer Academic Publishers. Printed in the Netherlands.

These responses result in the classical triad of signs in focal infection, heat, swelling and redness (rubor).

Despite many different methods which are used to try and inactivate ad destroy invading micororagnisms the loss of one or any of these factors can have a significant effect on the patient's ability to fight infection. For example in Chronic Granulomatous Disease patients without effective compliment are able to phagocytose but not destroy invading micro-organisms. This results in severe and debilitating granuloma forming at sites were infection is found but not eradicated. In patients with loss of immunoglobulin various syndromes can exist. However the absence of all immunoglobulin often ensures that death from overwhelming infection within the first five years of life unless the patient has a bone marrow transplant. Until recently the most common cause of these immunodeficiencies were hereditary and as a consequence rare. There are however some forms of acquired immunodeficiency. The most common cause being viral infection. In the influenza pandemic of 1918-1920 most deaths were from secondary pulmonary infections which occurred 1-3 weeks after the influenza infection became apparent. To a milder degree it is know that the Epstein -Barr virus, which causes infectious mononucleosis can lead to a temporary and normally inconsequential immunosuppression.

Acquired Immunosuppression.

Of more importance to all hospital physicians however has been the advance in the spread of a new retrovirus named the Human Immunodeficiency Virus (HIV). Since its early origins in Subsaharan Africa it has spread worldwide so that in 1990 11 million people were thought to be infected. The virus is lymphophilic and lymphotoxic . Its particular host is the 'helper' T-lymphocyte which expresses the immunological marker CD4 . This lymphocyte is responsible in the identification and presentation of invading microorganisms to the rest of the immune system for destruction. A different class of T-lymphocyte expressing CD8 is described as a 'suppressor' cell. Its main task being to limit the extent of reaction against the invader, presumably to reduce collateral damage to normal tissues. In HIV infection the normal predominance of CD4 cells is reversed so that these become less common. From a normal level of about 800/ml they can fall below 200/ml. This then initiated a syndrome of acquired infections which can become increasingly severe and life threatening. It is also known that some tumours such as Kaposi's sarcoma and lymphoma become more common. This syndrome is known as the acquired immunodeficiency syndrome (AIDS). A similar condition has been seen in some patients treated to suppress the immune system to prevent rejection of transplanted organs. In particular those who have received anti-thyroid globulin (ATG) also have a marked reduction in their CD4 count. They appear to suffer from an AIDS like syndrome but fortunately in many patients is reverable with the cessation of the ATG therapy.

In many ways the problem of the immunosupressed patient is as a consequence of modern medicine. As we are able to transplant various organs that need long term immunosuppression more patients will be at risk of such problems. It is also clear that in many parts of the world the way medicine is practised, for example using blood products and multiple venipunctures with unsterilised equipment, has lead to the exposure of many thousands of people to HIV. As it can also be spread by blood, semen and other bodily fluids these infected people can then spread the infection to others for example by sexual contact. In terms of nuclear medicine these patients present special problems as they have incompetent immune systems. They will not produce an immune response to any infection and granulocyte involvement in sites of infection is limited. The use of radiolabelled granulocytes is these patients is therefore limited.

The severely ill patient with multi-organ failure.

Patients who are admitted to hospital with complex problems may have sepsis as cause for their admission or may gain sepsis within the hospital environment. In all cases the most severely ill patients will suffer from multi-organ failure. They will need constant support of their breathing and possibly circulation. In addition they may have liver or kidney failure. Patients may have had to attend surgery and as a consequence be on sedating and pain relieving drugs all of which will attenuate the patients symptoms and signs. Most of these patients will be immunocompetent but unable to mount a significantly good response to the infection to ensure survival. In some patients a septic syndrome of tachycardia, hypotension and renal failure can occur and unless the infection is correctly identified and treated death follows within 24-48 hours. In these patients time is most important and nuclear medicine techniques must be able to provide accurate and fast localisation of infection

The Guests.

In traditional teaching of microbiology microorganisms were dived into those who were pathogenic man and those who not pathogenic. A few organisms such as the protozoa *Pneumocystis carinii* are commonly found in the environment but only occasionly caused disease in man. However the AIDS epidemic was discovered when 3 years stock of the drug Pentamidine used to treat *Pneumocystis carinii* was used up in 3 months.

Subsequent epidemiological investigations uncovered the new syndrome AIDS.

Patients can also have bizarre effects from known pathogens. *Candida albicans* a yeast which inhabits the skin can cause septesaemia in patients with AIDS. All these problems of abnormal hosts (the immunosupressed patient) and different hosts mean that nuclear medicine techniques may need to be adapted to this group.

Pulmonary Infections

Pulmonary infection with *Pneumocystis carinii* pneumonia (PCP) or other pathogens remains the major cause of death and morbidity in patients with AIDS (1). Whilst early recognition of this disease by better understanding of the radiological features (2) has improved over the years the mainstay of treatment remains empirical administration of high dose Co- trimoxazole and Pentamidine to all patients with AIDS who present short of breath. This treatment is unpleasant and can itself be immunosuppressive. There is some need to find a way to more accurately identify those patients with PCP. Planar chest X-rays can be negative in up to 40% of patients with early disease. Resolution of chest X-ray after treatment is variable especially if other lung disease such as Kaposi's sarcoma is present. Though it may be possible to identify *Pneumocystis* in the sputum by direct microcopy and polymerase chain reaction (PCR) in some patients lung biopsy via bronchoscopy and open lung biopsy may be needed.

A simple screening methods uses the washout rates from a Tc-99m diethyltripentaacetic acid (DTPA) aerosol which can be administered and imaged in about 20 minutes (3). The Tc-99m DTPA is removed by clearance from the main airways by transport with bronchial mucous. Once the Tc-99m DTPA has reached the alveolar it is transported across the alveolar membrane and cleared from the systemic circulation via the kidneys. In the simplest method the patient is supine and inhales the Tc-99m DTPA as an aerosol of particles of 1um diameter. Images are then obtained for up to 60 minutes. Regions of interest are drawn around each lung and a time activity curve of washout calculated.

If the washout is rapid and biexponential then the probability of PCP is high as the positive predictive value of the test is close to 90% (4). The test may also be of use in monitoring the effect if therapy as the washout curve returns to a slow mono-exponential curve after successful treatment for the PCP. However it can be non-specific and the washout rate can be abnormal in patients with a alveolitis due to infection or other causes such as after Bleomycin chemotherapy or other lung infections. It has been suggested however that if the chest-X-ray is normal and PCP is thought likely then the first line use of a Tc-99m DTPA aerosol is ideal. Patients with a negative study would then be considered for bronchoscopy and possibly a gallium-67 citrate study. Those with a positive study would be treated for PCP and only reinvestigated if they did not clinically improve.

Ga-67 Citrate.

The use of gallium-67 citrate (Ga-67) scintigraphy in AIDS has a history almost as long as the disease. In PCP there was diffuse uptake of Ga-67 citrate throughout both lungs (5-7). This pattern was felt to be almost diagnostic of PCP, though it now known that other diseases such as pneumococcal pneumonia and *mycobacterium avium intracellulare* infection can have a similar appearance (8). It was also noted that patients with Kaposi's sarcoma did not have uptake of Ga-67 citrate and therefore as both conditions can appear with similar symptoms and signs a positive Ga-67 citrate study will signify the presence of PCP. However to use the Ga-67 study just for this alone would be to reduce its effectiveness as a diagnostic tool. In many patients with AIDS symptoms and signs are non-specific. The patient may present with mild fever, unproductive cough, chest tightness and dyspnoea. Chest X-ray is either normal or non-specifically abnormal. The Ga-67 citrate image will therefore allow identification of a wide range of infections. Focal lymph node uptake is seen both in *mycobacterium tuberculosis* infection and in lymphoma. Focal lung uptake of Ga-67 citrate tends to suggest focal bacterial or fungal lung infection though in a few patients this can be the pattern seen with PCP. This appears to be secondary to partial treatment of PCP with nebulised Pentamidine leaving small pockets of peripheral alveolar untreated. *Mycobacterium avium intracellulare* infection which is now a major problem in patient with AIDS was thought to present with diffuse lung and lymph node uptake (Fig 2). However the pattern of abnormalities is much wider than previously seen with no specific patterns of abnormal uptake seen (8). Fig.1.

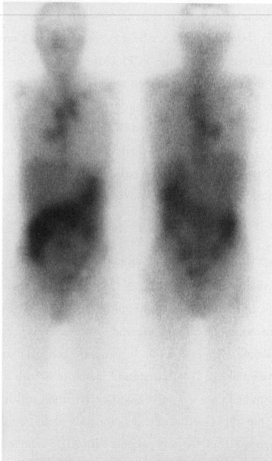

ANTERIOR WB   POSTERIOR WB

Figure 1. *Anterior and posterior whole body images of a patient with AIDS and Mycobacterium avium intracellulare infection demonstrating classical lymph node uptake of Gallium-67 citrate in the mediastinium and hilum. Note non-specific intense colonic uptake.*

It is important to note that when imaging patients with AIDS the Ga-67 scan may be suggestive but is often not diagnostic of a particular diagnosis..

It has been suggested that the specificity of Ga-67 imaging in the chest of AIDS patients can be increased from 20%-80% by only using activity as intense as the liver as pathological. (9). However this would reduce the sensitivity in finding pulmonary infections such as cytomegalovirus (CMV) where lung uptake is often less intense than liver uptake.

Labelled Leukocytes.

The lack of specificity of Ga-67 in being able to differentiate infection from other pathologies such as lymphoma led to attempts to use this technique in patients with AIDS. It was found that while there was a slight improvement in the sensitivity of labelled leukocytes over Ga-67 in localising infection in patients with AIDS the opposite was true in the chest were Ga-67 was superior (11,12). There are further worries with the technique as it requires extensive handling of blood products. This could lead to needle stick injury or splash contamination of the eyes with HIV infected blood. Even if it is possible using sealed cabinets to reduce this risk there is the possibility of maladministration of the labelled leukocytes from an HIV infected patient to one without HIV. This danger may be increased if a central blood labelling lab handling up to 100 blood samples a day is used. One attempt to avoid this problem has been the use of donated ABO combatable leukocytes (12). In this method leukocytes are separated form whole blood available in the hospital blood bank. After labelling they are injected in to the patient with AIDS. This technique has been shown to work in patients with bony and soft tissue infection but there is no published evidence that it will work in chest infections such as PCP. Alternative methods include the use of in vitro labelling via a radiolabelled anti-granulocyte antibody. This has been done using an antibody directed against the 250kDalton glycoprotein on the surface of the granulocyte (Tc-99m BW 250/183). Though only a number of patients have been studied the results are equally disappointing to those seen with autologous labelled leukocytes (13).

Why do such methods fail in the profoundly immunosupressed is because the guest organisms are often very different from those seen in the immunocompetent. *Pneumocystis carinii* very rarely induces any form of inflammatory response until late in the disease and granulocyte involvement is limited. The mycobacterium similarly may have some early granulocyte involvement but in its chronic form the infiltration is mainly lymphocytic. Whilst it is possible to label lymphocytes preferentially with either In-111 oxime or Tc-99m HMPAO after they have been separated from the granulocytes their survival is limited and it is unclear whether they could be used to image. Other methods of labelling T-lymphocytes in vivo include using monoclonal antibodies and interleukin-2. Neither agent has been used in patients with AIDS and suspected mycobacterial disease. The ideal agent then for imaging chest infections in the immunosupressed does not depend on granulocyte kinesis to the site of infection but is more specific than Ga-67.

Polyclonal IgG.

Polyclonal human immunoglobulin (HIG) is a non-specific agent which can be used to identify a wide variety infections (14,15). Initial work in patients with AIDS used a Tc-99m labelled HIG. It was found that whilst the results were similar in peripheral tissues it was inferior to Ga-67 in the chest and abdomen (16) . This was thought to be due to the high blood pool with this agent which was still significant at 24 hours post injection and due to the short 6 hour half life of the Tc-99m imaging beyond this time was not practical. It was felt that indium-111 may provide a better radiolabel allowing imaging out to 72 hours if required. In-111 HIG was compared with In-111 leukocytes in a series of 35 immunosupressed patients with fever but who were HIV negative. The In-111 HIG was able to find 6 more sites of infection than those seen with the labelled leukocytes (17). The In-111 HIG was able to see the site of infections caused by organisms such as fungi and viruses which are not normally visualised by labelled leukocytes and in pulmonary infection preceded changes seen on X-ray by 2-3 days. In-111 however is not an ideal isotope for imaging; its physical characteristics are less than ideal. Its long half life means that only limited activity can be given resulting in extended imaging time and poor count statistics. It is cyclotron produced and is expensive (74MBq -2mCi costing about $150) and is not readily available; and not available at all outside Europe and North America. For this reason it was thought that Tc-99m-HIG may be useful in patients with AIDS. However in a direct comparison with Ga-67 in 25 patients with AIDS presenting as a fever the sensitivity of the Tc-99m-HIG was only 55% and 8 sites of pulmonary infection found with Ga-67 the Tc-99m-HIG was negative (16). The reason for the low sensitivity of these patients was that there was persistent blood pool activity in the lungs and heart which did not clear before the images at 24 hours. Later images were not possible due to the 6 hour physical half life of the Tc-99m.

In-111 HIG was then applied to a group of AIDS patients presenting with suspected chest infection. In all cases in which pulmonary infection was subsequently proven there was abnormal uptake of the In-111 HIG (18). The pattern of uptake was also interesting in that diffuse uptake in both lungs was most commonly seen in PCP. Less intense diffuse pulmonary uptake of In-111 HIG was also seen in *Mycobacterium avium intracellulare* infection and cytomegalovirus pneumonitis. Focal uptake was seen in patients with a bacterial pneumonia. There were two cases of false positive uptake seen one in a patient with focal uptake in a chest haematoma following the patient being stabbed 10 days before the scan and another with end stage renal failure. There was no uptake in either Kaposi's sarcoma or lymphoma. The lack of uptake in lymphoma was of particular use as it is often a differential diagnosis of the cause of fever in patients with AIDS. So unlike Ga-67, In-111 HIG can differentiate between infection and lymphoma. It had been noted that in some non-AIDS patients with inflammatory lymphoma there was uptake of In-111 HIG. This is not a problem in patients with immunodeficiency as they are unable to raise an inflammatory response to the presence of the lymphoma.

It was also shown that the sensitivity for finding infection in 63 patients with AIDS was 97% with a specificity of 95%. Planar chest radiology had a sensitivity of 62% and a specificity of 43% (18). This means that the specificity of spinning a coin is better than planar radiology in AIDS patients with suspected chest infection.

Other Agents.

One agent which may be of particular use in the patient with known chest pathology is the thallium-201 chloride. When combined with a Ga-67 citrate image low grade uptake of thallium-201 chloride appears to be diagnostic of mycobacterial disease (19). Intense uptake occurs in Kaposi's sarcoma (Table 1).

Pathology	Gallium-67 citrate	Thallium-201 chloride
Pulmonary infection	Positive	Negative
Kaposi's sarcoma	Negative	Positive
Mycobacterial infection	Strongly positive	Weakly positive

Table 1 Patterns of uptake in the lungs of patients with AIDS using Gallium-67 citrate and Thallium-201 chloride

Another unique approach with micro-organism specific antibody directed against *Pneumocystis carinii* has been used to image 16 patients with suspected pneumonia . Six of these patients were subsequently found to have PCP (20). There was one false negative study in a partially treated patient and one false positive report in a patient with a mixture of pulmonary tuberculosis and Candida. This suggests it may be possible to identify if a patient has a specific infection. However what is less clear is how it will be possible to decide which patients should have such an organism specific study. This type of approach may be more useful in monitoring therapy than in diagnosis so that it will be possible to know when antimicrobials can be stopped. This will be of particular use in patients with multiple pathologies where it is important to know which medication can be terminated.

Conclusion: Pulmonary Infection.

At present there are only three methods available for imaging infection in the chest which are widely licenced. These are the Tc-99m DTPA aerosol, Ga-67 citrate and labelled leukocyte. As the sensitivity and specificity of labelled leukocytes in these patients is so low they should not be used if chest infection is suspected. Ideally if the chest X-ray is normal the patient should have a Tc-99m DTPA aerosol lung clearance study. If this is positive the patient should be treated for *Pneumocystis carinii* pneumonia. If the patient does not respond or has an abnormal chest X-ray the patient should have a Ga-67 citrate scan. If Kaposi's sarcoma is suggested by the chest X-ray or is known to be present in the lungs a sequential Tl -201 and Ga-67 citrate imaging protocol should be used. In-111 HIG may prove to be superior to Ga-67 citrate in both sensitivity and specificity however its commercial exploitation remains in question. If it becomeswidely available it should replace Ga-67 citrate in these patients. Ga-67 citrate would still have a useful role in the diagnosis of AIDS related lymphoma.

Patients with Fever of unknown origin.

Many patients with AIDS present not with specific symptoms with localising symptoms but with the triad of non-specific symptoms of fever, malaise and anorexia. In these patients repeat investigations using CT or ultrasound are often unhelpful and fail to identify the cause of the illness. The situation is not helped by the fact that HIV itself can lead to fever in the absence of other pathogens. Tumours such as lymphoma and Kaposi's sarcoma can present as fever. Also patients with AIDS are not 'immune' from the many other non-infective causes of fever.

Whilst Ultrasound and CT are useful in investigating the patient with AIDS and immunosuppression presenting with fever of unknown cause they have two distinct disadvantages. Firstly they rely on disruption of the normal anatomy. Whilst this may occur in many patients it may be less likely in immunosupressed individuals as the bodies inflammatory reaction is attenuated. Secondly both ultrasound and CT are regional studies. It is difficult to perform whole body CT and ultrasound is of limited use in the chest. For both these reasons it may useful to use a technique which easily images the whole body then allowing areas of abnormality to be identified for further investigation and biopsy (Fig 2).

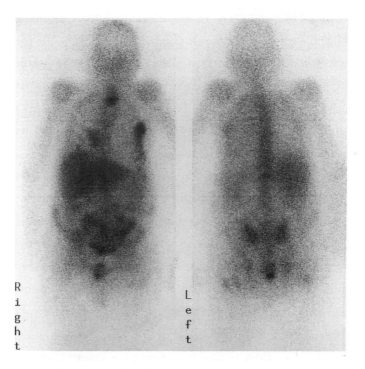

Figure 2. *Anterior and posterior whole body Gallium-67 citrate images of a patient post liver transplant with fever. Images demonstrate multiple sites of infection in the chest, these were subsequently found to be due to multiple staphylococcal abscesses.*

One such test is the Ga-67 citrate study. As described earlier, this test has been shown to be higher sensitive for the investigation of patients with immunosuppression and infection (7). However there are problems. The physiological distribution of Ga-67 citrate includes the gut, a major source of infection in the immunosupressed. In patients with AIDS high levels of colonic activity of Ga-67 citrate have been seen not only in gut infection but in those with generalised infection such as disseminated atypical mycobacterial disease and lymphoma (15). White cell imaging has been found to have a higher specificity than Ga-67 citrate. However as the sensitivity in the chest is so low it cannot be recommended in those patients who have no localising symptoms or signs as possible pulmonary infection may be missed. It has been suggested that early (4 hour) Ga-67 citrate imaging is more specific in the abdomen that later (>24 hour imaging) (21). The theory being that colonic excretion occurs after 24 hours therefore uptake in the gut before this time must be pathological. The high blood pool activity at 4 hours making interpretation of the images difficult. In a comparison of In-111 HIG, and Ga-67 in 25 patients with fever of unknown origin in patients with AIDS the sensitivity of the Ga-67 and In-111 was 90%, the specificity of the In-111 HIG was 87% compared to 65% for Ga-67 citrate (22). The largest number of false positive images seen involved colonic uptake in patients without colonic infection. It has been suggested that bowel purgatives may be of use. However in AIDS there is often significant bowel motility problems secondary to direct infection and destruction of the gut neurones by the HIV.

It would seem therefore that In-111 HIG may be the ideal agent in the immunosupressed (16) However the lack of a commercially available product will limit its widespread use. Therefore Ga-67 citrate scintigraphy remains the agent of choice in these patients. However there are less clear patterns of uptake than in imaging just the chest. For example it was thought that *Mycobacterium avium intracellulare* infection occurred if there was uptake of Ga-67 citrate within the extra-thoracic lymph nodes. This is only one presentation however and a wide range of abnormalities can be seen in patients with *Mycobacterial avium intracellulare* (Table 2)

It was found that if at least three of the above were present then the patient had a 89% likelihood of having *Mycobacterium avium intracellulare* (9).

Despite the fact that Ga-67 citrate scintigraphy is not ideal it is probably the best agent we

Site of abnormality on Ga-67 citrate scintigraphy (* greater than expected physiological activity)	Frequency (%)
Lung	39%
Extra thoracic lymph nodes	50%
Lacrimal*	44%
Parotid	22%
Colonic*	72%
Nasal sinus*	67%
Reduced activity in the bone marrow	55%

Table 2 pattern of abnormalities seen on Ga-67 citrate scintigraphy in 18 patients with *Mycobacterium avium intracellulare* infection

have available in patients who are immunosupressed. Improved localisation around the liver and the abdomen can be achieved by tomography. This can be achieved quickly using a two or three headed gamma camera. Liver subtraction techniques may also be of use in patients with suspected liver or sub-phrenic abscess. Whilst this is rare in patients with AIDS it is not uncommon following liver transplantation.

However the main problem with Ga-67 citrate is that it is often not considered until the patient has had many other investigations. In a review of the effectiveness of Ga-67 citrate in patients with AIDS it was found that Ga-67 citrate was ordered late in the patient's management (23).. Some patients waited 6 months after the onset of symptoms before the Ga-67 citrate scan was ordered. Not surprisingly in those patients in which the Ga-67 citrate study was ordered within 4 weeks of the onset of symptoms the scan had significantly more impact on the management of the patient than those with a greater than 4 week delay in ordering.

The message therefore seems to be that Ga-67 citrate imaging should be a first line investigation in the immunosupressed with fever but without localising signs. The results of the Ga-67 citrate study should then be used to guide ultrasound or CT. In the future it may be possible to replace Ga-67 citrate with either In-111 HIG or hopefully a Tc-99m labelled product.

Other Scintigraphic Tests used in the Immunocompromised.

A second approach to imaging infection is not to use agents such as Ga-67 citrate or labelled leukocytes to localise infection but look at the effect the infection has on the target organ.

For example HIV is neurotoxic and a significant proportion of patients suffer from a dementia type illness related to low grade encephalopathy (HIV encephalopathy). It is possible to use cerebral perfusion studies to help in the diagnosis of this condition. Using both F-18 flourodeoxyglucose (FDG) positron emission tomography (PET) or Tc-99m hexamethylprponyl amine oxime (HMPAO) single photon emission tomography (SPET) (24,25). In both cases there is a marked reduction of cerebral perfusion in the medial temporal lobes, followed by reduced perfusion in the frontal and posterior parietal lobes. These changes have been noted before the onset of clinical symptoms.. Also within the brain patient with significant T lymphocyte immunosuppression either from HIV or the administration of anti-T-lymphocyte globulin (ATG) can suffer a primary cerebral lymphoma or toxoplasmosis. Whilst toxoplasmosis tends to be multi focal and lymphoma uni focal there is significant overlap and CT or MRI may be unhelpful. It has again been demonstrated that thallium-201 chloride is very useful in differentiating these two pathologies. The uptake in primary cerebral lymphoma is approximately 7 times that of normal brain tissue or brain infected with toxoplasmosis (26). Therefore any suspicious intra cerebral lesion seen on CT or MRI in a immunosupressed patient should result in a Thallium-201 SPET study.

Another common area of infection is the biliary system. Cholangitis with sclerosis is common in patients with AIDS and in some cases can become symptomatic. Ultrasound is helpful only in advanced cases. Both CT and hepatobiliary scintigraphy provide a sensitive method (90%) with which to find the presence of AIDS related sclerosing cholangitis (27).

Finally it must not be forgotten that simple tests such as the dynamic bone scintigraphy for suspected bone and joint infection have a role to play in these patients.

Severely ill patients with multiple organ failure

The emphasis for the investigation of the severely ill patient is often different than with the immunosupressed. There may be significant localising symptoms or signs. There is a need to find the correct answer with accuracy and alacrity. The typical Ga-67 citrate imaging regime of imaging at 72 hours is not appropriate for the acutely sick patient where time may be essential to save lives. Symptoms and signs may also be confusing as the patient may have significant preceding pathology or be post surgical. For example a patient with abdominal pain after a laparotomy could have post surgical pain but more sinister pathology such as a post surgical infection may be present.

When the diagnosis is not apparent than simple investigations are required both planar X-ray and ultrasound should be used as they are cheap and available at the patient's bed side. If these prove to be unhelpful then second line investigations such as CT or scintigraphic infection imaging must be considered. If there are localising signs then CT is to be recommended as it will enable any sites of infection to br biopsies and if pyogenic for the pus to be removed for culture and microscopy. However in those patients with no localising signs then the a nuclear medicine study should be considered. The main studies available are listed in Table 3.

It has been shown that to develop a service in which scintigraphic techniques are used it is essential to provide a rapid response to the clinician's's request (28). In practice this means that only Tc-99m labelled agents be considered appropriate. Therefore as the only agent with sufficient sensitivity and specificity is Tc-99m HMPAO labelled leukocytes, these should be used in the acutely ill patient. It is possible using standard imaging techniques and imaging at 1 and 3 hours post re injection of labelled leukocytes to provide clinically useful answers within 5-6 hours of the request being made.

Whilst many clinicians may be reluctant to let their patient travel to the nuclear medicine department, this same attitude is not normally expressed if the patient is to have a CT or MRI. It is however normally possible using mobile ventilators and the assistance of an intensive care physician and nurse to transport a patient safely to and from nuclear medicine. The open gantry of most nuclear medicine cameras also means that imaging can be simpler and most pillar and stand nuclear medicine cameras are able to move in such a way that anterior images are possible with the patient on their own bed. These may prove to be sufficient. In all cases close co-operation between staff of both nuclear medicine and

Agent	Advantages	Disadvantages
Ga-67 citrate	Readily available	Imaging needed for 72 hours Expensive Normal bowel excretion
In-111 labelled leukocytes	High sensitivity and specificity Good images 4 and 24 hours	Cell labelling facilities needed Expensive Poor availability
Tc-99m HMPAO labelled leukocytes	Isotope readily available High sensitivity and specificity Imaging in abdomen finished by 3.5 hours	Cell labelling facilities required HMPAO expensive
Tc-99m HIG	Isotope readily available Good sensitivity and specificity in periphery Rapid imaging	High renal and blood pool activity means it cannot be used in abdomen or chest
In-111 HIG	Good sensitivity Good specificity	Imaging needed at 24 and 48 hours Isotope not readily available Expensive No commercial preparation
Tc-99m nanocolloid	Isotope readily available Imaging finished in 1.5 hours	Does not seem to work!

Table 3.[opposite]. *Advantages and disadvantages of different agents used to image infection.*
the intensive therapy unit should ensure no significant practical problems.

Accuracy of scintigraphic imaging of infection in the severely ill patient.

Whilst no direct comparison have been published in this patient group alone there is data
supporting the use of nuclear medicine techniques in patients with focal infection some of
whom are acutely ill. In a series of 25 patients presenting either with fever and acute
abdominal pain or post-operative fever Tc-99m HMPAO labelled leukocytes were able to
identify all 76% of all abscesses whilst ultrasound found 71% of abscesses. However the
labelled leukocyte studies did not find four liver abscesses which could have been found in
liver subtraction had been performed. If extra-hepatic abscesses only are counted then the
sensitivity of Tc-99m HMPAO leukocytes was 100% but ultrasound only 62 %. In both
cases there were no false positive labelled leukocyte studies but specificity of ultrasound was
only 87% (29). The authors clearly feel that nuclear medicine was superior to ultrasound
in these patients. If they performed liver subtraction techniques which is obligatory in all
acutely ill patients they would have even more impressive data. Similar results were
obtained when Gallium-67 citrate was compared with ultrasound (30). The sensitivity of
gallium-67 citrate was 92% in acute abdominal infection whilst ultrasound sensitivity was
60% (Fig 3).

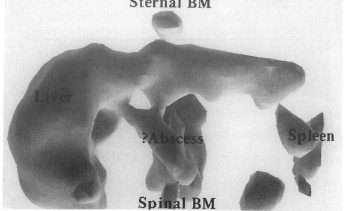

Figure 3. *Three dimensional display of Gallium-67 SPET in a post surgical patient showing
abnormal uptake below the liver. Inferior view 3D image. This was confirmed as an abscess
on CT*

What we do not have data on however is how nuclear medicine techniques compare with CT. This may be particularly important as the speed of the new third generation spiral CTs combined with the acquisition of contiguous data makes CT both more accurate and also more available to the severely ill patient.

Of the techniques currently available for imaging infection the speed at which answers are required really limits the nuclear physician to either Tc-99m labelled leukocytes or using a Tc-99m labelled anti-granulocyte antibody (31) to label granulocytes in vivo. With both agents a clinically relevant answer should be available within 6 hours of the request (Fig 4).

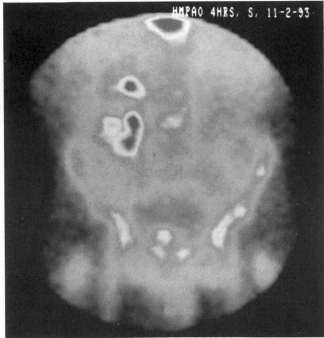

Figure 4. *Patient 72 hours post surgery for appendix abscess. Images 4 hours post reinjection of Tc-HMPAO white cells show intense uptake in the right side of the abdomen. This was found to be due to multiple abscesses on repeat laparotomy performed 1 hour after this image was acquired.*

The most important thing however is to consider the early use of scintigraphic techniques in these patients. Therefore as soon as ultrasound or CT has failed to find a focus of infection in the critically ill patient with sepsis a nuclear medicine test should be initiated.

References

1. Peters BS, Beck EJ, Coleman DG, Wadsworth MJH, McGuiness O, Pinching AJ. Changing disease patterns in patients with AIDS in a referral centre in the United Kingdom: The changing face of AIDS. Br Med J 1991; 302, 203-206.
2. Naidich DP, Garay SM, Leitman BS, McCanley DI. Radiological manifestations of pulmonary disease in the acquired immunodeficiency syndrome (AIDS). Semin Roentol 1987; 42, 14-30.
3. O' Doherty MJ, Page CJ, Bradbeer CS et al. The place of Tc-99m DTPA aerosol transfer in the investigation of lung infections in HIV positive patients. Resp Med 1989; 83, 402-405.
4. Rosso J, Guillon JM, Parrot A et al. Technetium-99m-DTPA and Gallium-67 scanning in pulmonary complications of human immunodeficiency virus infection. J Nucl Med 1992; 22, 700-7.
5. Bitran J, Bekerman C, Weinstein R, Bennet C, Ryo U, Pinsky S. Patterns of gallium-67 scintigraphy in patients with acquired immune deficiency syndrome and AIDS related complex. J Nucl Med 1987; 28, 1103-1106.
6. Kramer EL, Sangar JH, Garay SM, et al Gallium-67 scans of the chest of patients with immunodeficiency. J Nucl Med 1987; 28, 1107-1114.
7. Kramer EL, Sangar JH, Garary SM, Grossman RJ, Tiu S, Banner H. Diagnostic implications of Ga-67 chest scan patterns in human immunodeficiency virus-seropositive patients Radiol 1989; 170, 671-677.
8. Buscombe JR, Buttery P, Ell PJ, Miller RF. Patterns of Ga-67 citrate accumulation in human immunodeficiency virus positive patients with and without *Mycobacterium avium intracellulare* infection Clin Radiol 1995; 50, 483-488.
9. Coleman DL, Hattner RS, Luce JM, Dodek PM, Golden JA, Murray JF. Correlation between gallium lung scans and fibre optic bronchoscopy in patients with suspected *Pneumocystis carinii* pneumonia, and the acquired immunodeficiency syndrome. Am Rev Respir Dis 1984; 130, 1166-1169.
10. Fineman DS, Palestro CJ, Kim CK. Detection of abnormalities in febrile AIDS patients with In-111 labeled leukocyte and Ga-67 scintigraphy. Radiol 1989; 170, 677-680.
11. Palestro CJ, Goldsmith SJ. The role of gallium and labelled leukocyte scintigraphy in the AIDS patient. Q J Nucl Med 1995; 39, 221-230.
12. O' Doherty MJ, Revell P, Page CJ, Lee S, Mountford MJ, Nunan TO. Donor leucocyte imaging in patients with AIDS: A preliminary report. Eur J Nucl Med 1990; 17, 327-333.
13. Prulovich EM, Miller RF, Costa DC et al. Immunoscintigraphy with a Tc-99m labelled antigranulocyte antibody in patients with human immunodeficiency virus infection and AIDS. Nucl Med Commun 1995; 10, 838-845.
14. Fishman AJ, Rubin RH, Khaw BA et al. Detection of acute inflammation with In-111 labeled non-specific polyclonal IgG Semen. Nucl Med 1988; 18, 335-344.
15. Buscombe J, Oyen WAG, Corstens FHM. Use of polyclonal IgG in HIV infection and AIDS. Q J Nucl Med 1995; 39, 212-220.
16. Buscombe J, Lui D, Miller RF, Ell PJ. Combined Ga-67 citrate and Tc-99m human immunoglobulin imaging in patients infected with the human immunodeficiency virus (HIV). Nucl Med Commun 1991; 12, 583-592.
17. Oyen WJG, Claessens RAMJ, Raemaekers JMM, De Pauw BE, van der Meer JWM, Cortsens FHM. Diagnosing infection in febrile granulocytopaenic patients with indium-111 labeled human immunoglobulin. J Clin Oncol 1992; 10, 61-68.
18. Buscombe J, Oyen WAG, Corstens FHM, Ell PJ, Miller RF. A comparison of In-111 HIG scintigraphy and chest radiology in the identification of pulmonary infection of patients with HIV

infection. Nucl Med Commun 1995; 16, 327-335.

19. Abdel - Dayem HM, Bag R, Macapinlac H, Elgazzar AH, Habbab N, Pescatore F, Kempf J. Diffuse Tl -201 uptake in the lungs. Etiologic classification and pattern recognition. Clin Nucl Med 1995; 20, 164-172 .

20. Goldenberg DM, Sharkey RM, Udem S. et al. Immunoscintigraphy of *Pneumocystis carinii* pneumonia in AIDS patients. J Nucl Med 1994; 35, 1028-1034.

21. Sanchez J, Mohannadi S, Kampf J, Singh M, Kaufman D, Abdel - Dayem H. Significance of early 4 hours gallium bowel activity in AIDS population. *In* Proceedings of the 5th Asia and Oceania Congress of Nuclear Medicine and Biology, Jakarta, Indonesia, 1992; 171 .

22. Buscombe J, Oyen WAG, Corstens FHM, Ell PJ, Miller RF. Localization of infection in HIV antibody positive patients with fever. Comparison of Ga-67 citrate and Radiolabelled human IgG. Clin Nucl Med 1995; 20, 334-339.

23. Wassie E, Buscombe J, Miller RF, Ell PJ. Gallium-67 citrate scintigraphy in AIDS; a clinical audit of its usefulness. Br J Radiol 1994; 67, 349-352.

24. Rottenberg DA, Moellar J, Stotler SC, et al. The metabolic pathology of AIDS dementia complex. Ann Neurol 1987; 22, 700-706.

25. Kramer EL, Sanger JJ. Brain imaging in the acquired immunodeficiency syndrome dementia complex. Sem Nucl Med 1990; 20, 353-363.

26. Dierckx RA, Martin JJ, Dobbeleir A, Crols R, Neetens I, De Deyn PP. Sensitivity and specificity of thallium-201 single-photon emission tomography in the functional detection and differential diagnosis of brain tumours. Eur J Nucl Med 1994; 21, 621-633.

27. Buscombe J, Miller RF, Ell PJ. The role of hepatobiliary scintigraphy in the diagnosis of AIDS related sclerosing cholangitis. Nucl Med Commun 1992; 13, 154-160.

28. Childs J, Buscombe J, Marshall D, Ryan P. Using clinical audit and algorithms in the scintigraphic imaging of infection. J Nucl Med Technol 1995; 23, 262-266.

29. Weldon MJ, Joseph AEA, French A, Saverymutu SH, Maxwell JH. Comparison of Technetium-99m - HMPAO labelled leucocyte and Indium-111- tropolonate labelled granulocytes and ultrasound in the diagnosis of intr-abdominal abscess. Gut 1995; 37, 557-564.

30. Lisbona R, Cassof J, Angtuaco E, Satin R. Comparative accuracy and complimentary use of Ga-67 citrate imaging and ultrasound in the diagnosis of abdominal disease. Clin Nucl Med 1979; 4, 108-110.

31. Becker W, Sapintogino A, Wolf F. Diagnostic accuracy of a late single technetium-99m-antigranulocyte antibody scan in inflammatory or infectious diseases. J Nucl Med 1991; 32, 1002.

CHAPTER 8

INFLAMMATORY BOWEL DISEASE

Michael J. Weldon

Introduction

Inflammatory bowel disease (IBD) is a chronic condition with a relapsing course which often begins at an early age and affects the patient for life. It involves the bowel to a variable extent. In ulcerative colitis (UC) it is limited to the colon whereas in Crohn's disease it can affect any part of the bowel, in a discontinuous fashion. Management depends on knowledge of the type, site, extent and activity of inflammation and in Crohn's disease, other aspects of the disease contributing to severity such as fistulation, abscesses and malabsorption [1]. Because of the need for repeated investigation of the patient, the least invasive approach is desirable. Such approaches will be discussed in this chapter in addition to investigation of suspected complicating intra-abdominal sepsis.

Disease extent

The extent assessment need not be exact in routine clinical practice but an accurate assessment of the total degree of inflammation is needed particularly in therapeutic trials. The place where barium studies have a particular role is in the detection and evaluation of anatomical complications of IBD such as strictures, fistulae and carcinoma in advanced cases [1]. However, studies comparing barium enema assessment with post-operative examination of the resected specimen [2] demonstrated underestimation of extent using barium. A further consideration is the radiation dose which is variable but approximately 7-10 mSv which is not negligible considering that Crohn's disease patients may need several studies [1]. Colonoscopy provides direct visualisation and histology; however, incomplete examination may occur due to technical difficulties, or stricturing. Both colonoscopy and barium radiology are invasive and may be unpleasant for the patient. A less invasive approach is therefore needed.

Various radioisotope methods have been used over the years to image inflammation. The

P. H. Cox and J. R. Buscombe (eds.), The Imaging of Infection and Inflammation, 161–182.

behaviour of neutrophils within the body and their localisation in pathological processes has been a subject of study since the late 19th century [3]. Early studies used radioactive tracers to study this behaviour. They were unsuitable for external detection as they were not efficient gamma emitters. It was therefore not possible to study the in vivo kinetics and distribution of the labelled cells [4].

67-Gallium-citrate, a gamma emitter which accumulates at sites of infection, inflammation and neoplasia was then used producing positive images [5]. This isotope has a long half life which limits the dose that can be administered. The mechanism of uptake at the above sites involves binding to transferrin and lactoferrin at the site of pathology. However the technique was found to lack both sensitivity and specificity and posed difficulties in interpretation due to intestinal excretion. However it remains the most useful test in pyrexia of unknown origin since it also detects non inflammatory causes such as lymphoma [5].

Although IBD is a chronic disease with a predominantly mononuclear infiltrate, intense neutrophil recruitment is a feature common to both active Crohn's disease and ulcerative colitis (UC). This phenomenon has been used to advantage as a patient's own radiolabelled neutrophils migrate to sites of acute inflammation (as well as to bone marrow, liver and spleen). In 1976, 111-Indium labelled white cell scanning was introduced. This involved taking a sample of blood, labelling the white cells and reinjecting them into the patient and then gamma camera imaging [6]. Autoradiographic studies showed that the 111-Indium label remained attached to whole granulocytes in colonic fluid and mucosal brushings with cells in crypt abscesses by 110 minutes [7]. Various in vitro viability tests were performed on 111-Indium labelled neutrophils including random migration, and chemotaxis which were normal at the in vivo doses used [8]. However, many authors felt that the in vivo migration of labelled cells was the most sensitive index of cell viability. Damaged cells are quickly removed by the lung reticuloendothelial system resulting in persistent lung uptake beyond 20 minutes and higher liver activity than expected [9]. Several studies were carried out which demonstrated the accuracy of this technique in evaluating the extent of IBD 9. However, it has some limitations including the need to purify neutrophils for optimal results, relatively poor quality images due to the small quantity of radiation that can be administered because of the long half life of the isotope of 67 hours and limited hospital availability.

Attempts have therefore been made to replace 111-Indium with 99mTechnetium (Tc) with a half life of only 6 hours. In 1986 the first report of a lipophilic ligand; hexamethyl propylene amine oxine (HM-PAO) appeared [10]. Neirinckx and collaborators had succeeded in finding a hexamethyl derivative of propylene amine oxime (PAO). Two attractive features of this compound were, firstly, its ability to label cells in plasma enriched (20%) saline preserving viability and secondly, its relative stability in granulocytes compared with other blood cells [10]. 99mTc-HM-PAO is chemically unstable in the body and readily converts from its highly lipophilic primary form which allows it to cross cell membranes, to secondary hydrophilic species [11]. This conversion takes place rapidly in cells and various organs of the body. The rapid intracellular conversion to hydrophilic species that cannot diffuse across cell membranes explains its retention in the brain and white blood cells. The agent therefore effectively provides a pure granulocyte label without the necessity for granulocyte purification from a mixed leucocyte preparation. When used to image IBD, very high quality images are obtained (figure 1) and good correlations were found in an early clinical study with radiology, colonoscopy and surgery [12] and in subsequent studies [13]. It had the advantages of a simpler labelling technique, a lower radiation dose of only 3.3mSv, (this compares to approximately 7mSv for a 111-Indium scan and 0.05 mSv for a chest X-ray; the recommended maximum background radiation exposure to the general public per year is 5.0 mSv [14]) and high quality images. However, it suffers from renal excretion resulting in bladder and kidney images and is non specifically excreted into the colon particularly after 3 hours post injection.

In a comparison of the biodistribution of 99mTc-HMPAO with 111-Indium - tropolonate labelled granulocytes there was little difference in the clinical information provided by the two techniques [13]. A comparison of the kinetic characteristics of these techniques showed few differences [15].

In our own studies abdominal images were acquired 1 and and 3 hours after reinjection of radiolabelled leucocytes to show the extent of disease. Pelvic outlet views were required in order to image the rectum posteriorly, separately from the bladder anteriorly (figure 1). The 1 hr image gave the most accurate estimation of histological disease extent [16]. A large italian study of Crohn's disease reported a correlation of r = 0.85 for histological scoring and 0.65 for macroscopic appearances using visual scan grading. The poorer correlation with endoscopic appearances is not surprising as this is a poor indicator of disease activity [17]. Importantly the scan was negative in all 52 normal cases, in contrast to a smaller study [18] which reported false positives. The latter study used both 99mTc labelled colloid and 99mTc-HM-PAO and was of an odd design as many patients with positive images were not investigated and were dismissed on clinical grounds as unlikely to be true positives particularly patients being investigated for suspected abscesses. Moreover, not all possible IBD patients with positive images were investigated with histology. The validity of these results must therefore be brought into question. Sensitivity, specificity and predictive values should be given rather than false positive rate to be meaningful. In our experience, diffuse very low grade activity is occasionally seen particularly in the right iliac fossa or central abdomen after 2 hours. The configuration of this uptake does not conform to any particular bowel segment and is therefore easily distinguished from bowel mucosal activity as noted by other workers [19].

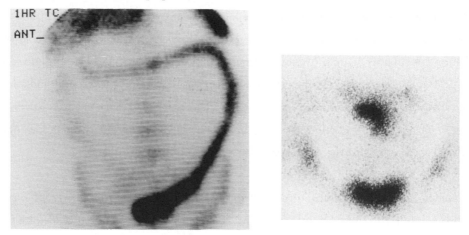

Figure 1. *99m Technetium-HM-PAO white cell scan showing bowel inflammation on anterior view (a) and inferior view (b) showing bladder activity anteriorly with rectal activity posteriorly*

Papos et al [20] reported sensitivity for detection of Crohn's disease of only 53% compared to 87% in UC. The reason for this becomes obvious as the histological findings in Crohn's disease were described as only a lymphocyte infiltrate. This suggests that largely inactive Crohn's disease was studied in which there was little neutrophil recruitment. This underlines the point that neutrophil scanning measures only active disease and this is its main application. Other studies found low sensitivity for the detection of Crohn's disease for the same reason [21]. This does not weaken the argument for excluding bowel inflammation in atypical cases of Irritable Bowel Syndrome (IBS), a non-inflammatory condition, [22] as patients are symptomatic at presentation with active disease permitting high sensitivity of disease detection e.g. 95% in one study [19]. 99mTc-HMPAO can accurately assess the extent of colonic disease in both Crohn's disease and ulcerative colitis (UC) by comparison with colonoscopic histology [16]. 99mTc-HMPAO has therefore replaced 111Indium as the isotope of choice for imaging acute intestinal inflammation [23].

All of these studies have relied largely on the correlation between the number of diseased segments and the number of segments with a positive scan. Provided that these segments are the same ones then the results are of value. No study has investigated in depth the segmental agreement. This is important as the site of disease will determine the mode of treatment. We used three statistical methods to examine agreement between histology and scanning for each of eight colonic segments in 58 patients Agreement using kappa statistics was high (table 1). It is important to realise that histological confirmation of the diagnosis in every case is crucial; documented positive white cell scans have been seen in necrotic colonic carcinoma 24, any form of colitis and lymphoma [25].

Other radio-isotope methods include direct labelling of human immunoglobulin with 99mTc [26] or 111-Indium. This however has not been successful due to non specific activity and very poor quality images [27]. A new approach is to use radiolabelled antigranulocyte antibodies [28]. This technique is still in its infancy and worries persist due to the use of murine antibodies. However developments in the "humanisation" of such antibodies may lead to a useful technique [29].

Other studies utilising the phagocytosis of radiolabelled stannous colloid have been reported [30]. Comparison with 111-Indium labelled leucocytes in 40 patients, 19 of whom had suspected IBD revealed 70% sensitivity. This low sensitivity was probably due to the very short half life of 99mTc colloid leucocytes in the circulation of 1.2hrs, most likely due to reticuloendothelial system uptake. The normal half-life of circulating neutrophils is 7 hours [13]. Several authors have expressed reservations about this method as phagocytosis results in cell activation and non physiological behaviour on re-injection [31]. Furthermore images only positive at 24hrs were interpreted as positive when it is known that by this time radiolabelled leucocytes have traversed the bowel mucosa into the lumen [25].

Differential diagnosis of colitis

Since the distribution of colitis differs between Crohn's disease and UC, and disease distribution is clearly demonstrated using 99mTc-HM-PAO (figure 2), we undertook a pilot study to assess its value in differential diagnosis in 38 consecutive patients with colitis and a positive scan. Using established features known to assist in distinction between these diseases i.e. rectal sparing, left sided disease, right sided disease, skip lesions, perianal disease and ileo-colonic disease, a simple visual scoring system was devised. The final clinical diagnosis based on all available clinical, radiological and histological information (but excluding the white cell scan) was 18 cases of UC and 20 of Crohn's colitis. Other diagnostic systems were also used to compare to the scan diagnosis as follows:- 1) Lennard-Jones criteria [32] based on results of investigations showing disease distribution, evidence of transmural disease, fibrosis and histological criteria; 2) OMGE (World Organisation of Gastroenterology) [33] based on clinical, radiological, endoscopic and histolological findings; 3) Colonoscopy score, [34] based only on macroscopic colonoscopy findings. There was very good agreement (92% with Lennard-Jones method) between the scan diagnostic criteria and all of the diagnostic systems used in this pilot study. The weakest agreement of 84% was with the macroscopic colonoscopy score which excluded histology and therefore was less accurate [16].

Disease Activity.

Various methods have been employed to measure the "activity" of IBD such as clinical scores, the acute phase response, and T cell activation studies such as circulating soluble IL-2 receptor levels. The most widely used method to assess Crohn's disease activity is the "Crohn's disease activity index" (CDAI) [35]. Such indices can be criticised because subjective elements such as well being and abdominal pain score have a considerable impact

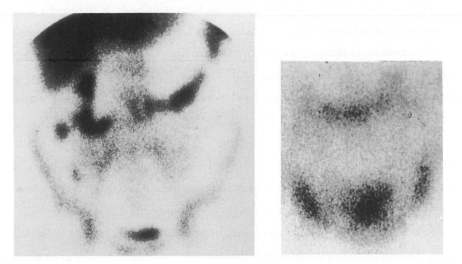

Figure 2. *99m Technetium-HMPAO white cell scan showing skip lesions and right sided disease on anterior view [a] and rectal sparing on inferior view[b] in a case of crohn's cholitis.*

which are influenced for example by the euphoriant effect of steroids [36], stress and by the personality of the patient; moreover, symptoms may be due to surgical complications, bowel frequency may be high for many non-inflammatory reasons e.g. post resection causing steatorrhea or bile salt diarrhoea. Clinical scores are therefore a better measure of illness or severity than a measure of bowel inflammation [37].

The enhanced release of cytokines is thought to amplify the immune response by recruiting neutrophils and mononuclear cells to the bowel by activating adhesion molecules. Such measures provide an insight into pathogenesis but are limited in the clinical assessment of individual patients. Measures of the associated acute phase response lack sensitivity and specificity [38]. Moreover, they fail to localise the site of active disease.

Colonoscopy and histological examination of mucosal biopsy specimens is regarded as the gold standard for the assessment of disease extent and activity in UC. Several endoscopic classifications appear to be useful for categorising patients as quiescent to severe UC [39].

Endoscopic assessment of Crohn's disease is much more difficult. It is a patchy disease; it can involve the small bowel and the frequency of strictures often limits access. A weighted, multiple regression analysis of the Crohn's Disease Endoscopic Index of Severity revealed poor correlation with clinical findings [40]. Furthermore mucosal biopsies have several drawbacks including accessibility in small bowel disease, their superficial nature and sampling error. Interobserver variation has also been found in some studies [41].

The uptake of radiolabelled neutrophils in bowel is a direct measure of bowel inflammation and therefore disease activity. Localisation of this active disease is important since some therapeutic agents such as enema preparations may only be suitable for distal colitis while the drug delivery systems of other agents may be better adapted for treating more proximal disease. An early, important finding was that after recruitment of radiolabelled white cells to the bowel during active disease, there is excretion of leucocytes into the bowel lumen. Measurement of the faecal excretion of labelled neutrophils over 4 days following injection was shown to be a more accurate method than scan interpretation of disease activity [42], although there was some dependency on frequency of defaecation in mild disease. Several studies have shown that 111-Indium labelled white cells can measure disease activity as accurately as colonoscopy and histology. A sensitivity of 97% for faecal 111-Indium granulocyte excretion and 94% for 111-Indium granulocyte scanning compared to 79% for radiology and 70% for rectal histology using colonoscopy with histology as reference standard has been reported [42]. An alternative, and much more practical method is the whole body retention of 111-Indium labelled white cells rather than measuring faecal loss to measure changes in disease activity [43].

However, quantitative 99mTc-HM-PAO scanning may surpass 111-Indium methods for several reasons including practicality and radiation dose. Faecal excretion estimations cannot be used to measure disease activity as there is colonic excretion of the isotope after 3-4 hours [13]. Visual assessment of 99mTc-HM-PAO scans provides a method of measuring activity as the physiological uptake in bone marrow, liver and spleen differs in increasing order allowing simple comparison with bowel uptake (figure 1) [16]. This method has been used with success in monitoring response to therapy [44]. Visual scoring appears satisfactory in the follow up of individual patients by the same clinician, but some studies have demonstrated interobserver variation [13], [45], with agreement on extent as low as 76% and activity, 78% 25. However this may depend on the scoring method since we have shown low interobserver variation as have others with agreement on extent of 94% and activity of 93% [9],[46]. On the whole, this method is rather crude and subjective. This does not limit its clinical use but more objective quantification is needed for therapeutic studies [9].

Improved objectivity can be provided by the use of computerised quantification of counts in the bowel which reflect neutrophil recruitment. A two dimensional

Segment	Observed Agreement	Chance Agreement	Kappa	Test of Agreement
A	98.13%	71.19%	0.9349	P<0.0001
B	98.30%	70.87%	0.9415	P<0.0001
C	97.92%	70.16%	0.9302	P<0.0001
D	97.55%	68.77%	0.9215	P<0.0001
E	93.86%	68.96%	0.8022	P<0.0001
F	95.18%	69.12%	0.8438	P<0.0001
G	94.83%	69.08%	0.8327	P<0.0001
H	94.40%	68.03%	0.8327	P<0.0001

Table 1. *Weighted Cohen's kappa assessment of agreement between 99m-Tc-HM-PAO scan and histology. Kappa > 0.8 denotes good agreement.*

method has been described in which all background activity is subtracted from the image leaving only bowel activity. An approximation for background activity has been used so far but "true" background subtraction is unlikely to be developed. This method has been used successfully to assess the response to therapy [45].

Single photon emission computerised tomography (SPECT) is a three dimensional imaging technique which has already proved useful in quantitative studies on blood flow in brain and heart [47]. Radioactive distributions in selected planes is clearly shown while the information from adjacent structures is blurred, minimised or absent. Moreover, by performing several transaxial scans through the abdomen, the complete three-dimensional distribution of radioactivity can be obtained and total bowel activity as well as individual segment activity in colon or small bowel can be measured. We used SPECT with 99mTc-HM-PAO to measure the neutrophil infiltrate in each colonic segment which correlated with the histological score for each segment [48]. Transaxial slices allowed clear separation of both lumbar spine marrow activity and bowel segment activity in both colon (figure 3) and in small bowel (figure 4). This method therefore offers the potential to measure changes in disease activity in different parts of the bowel in response to agents which may vary in their site of maximum delivery and action. Interestingly, patients requiring colectomy had very elevated total SPECT scores suggesting a method of detecting high risk patients in addition to the original indices described by Truelove and Witt's [49].

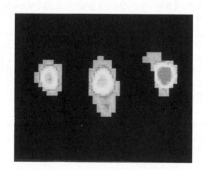

Figure 3. *Transaxial mid abdominal slice image from patient with total colitis showing ascending (left) and descending (right) colon and bone marrow activity (centre).*

Since the majority of labelled cells are granulocytes, purification of granulocytes before labelling with 99mTc-HMPAO is not necessary although it has recently been described [22]. SPECT has not yet been used in therapeutic trials but has now been refined to measure total colonic counts which reflect the total colonic neutrophil infiltrate. It has the advantages over older techniques of speed (results obtained within 3 hours, rather than 4 days) and both patient and technician acceptability (no need for stool analysis). Most gamma cameras currently in use in the U.K. are capable of performing SPECT imaging. While SPECT scanning is not required in routine clinical practice [50], accurate, objective evaluation of novel therapies for IBD is now possible using such techniques. The costs of 99mTc-HMPAO SPECT scanning must be set against the benefits of non-invasive location and measurement of inflammation, and the need to recruit fewer patients in trials where truly objective assessments are provided.

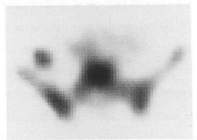

Figure 4. *Transaxial pelvic view showing terminal ileal Crohn's disease.*

Although Almer et al [51] showed no benefit from using a computerised technique compared to visual grading, others [45] demonstrated the superiority of their computerised method over planar imaging. Further experience of quantification techniques such as SPECT will be needed before the role of computerised quantification is clarified.

Small bowel disease

Using barium radiology, particularly the small bowel enema, it is possible to detect Crohn's disease at a very early stage, including such changes as distorted folds, which are thickened and contain aphthoid ulcers. The extent and features of Crohn's disease can be determined, as well as the presence of skip lesions [52]. While in former times, a barium study was performed to evaluate the functional state of the small bowel, nowadays, the recognition of morphological changes is the main aim [1]. Since histology is largely inaccessible, radio-labelled white cells provide a reasonable way to assess the neutrophil infiltrate and hence the degree of acute inflammation. Although the results of a preliminary study were encouraging using 111-Indium scanning [53], the small bowel was more difficult to image than large bowel because it is more mobile and transit is faster, resulting in blurring of images during the long acquisition time required for 111-Indium imaging. A previous study using 111-Indium mixed white cells found only a poor agreement on disease location with barium studies [54]. Other studies using 111-Indium white cells were 100% [53] and 72%

sensitive [55] in detecting disease. However, image quality was generally poor using 111-Indium. The intravenous use of glucagon has been used in order to suspend the movement of the bowel which has improved the clarity of images [56].

Our early experience quickly showed that good quality images could be obtained using 99mTc-HM-PAO [16]. Small bowel uptake was defined as a "tubular" configuration of uptake on 1 hour images outside the anatomical boundaries of the large bowel with transit into large bowel on 3 hour images. For example terminal ileal disease produced a very characteristic sigmoid appearance in the right iliac fossa on the one hour image with intraluminal transit into the ascending colon at three hours (figure 5) which distinguished it from a long loop of sigmoid colon producing transit into the rectum.

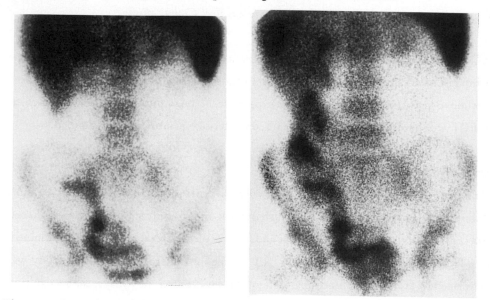

Figure 5. *Typical appearance of terminal ileal Crohn's disease on 1 hour (a) and 3 hour (b) 99m-Tc-HM-PAO scans.*

A previous retrospective study using 99mTc-HM-PAO showed good agreement with small bowel radiology and in fact provided extra information in two out of 18 patients [57]. Our study comparing small bowel meal appearances and 99mTc-HM-PAO scanning of 32 patients with suspected or known Crohn's disease was prospective and illustrated several points. Small bowel Crohn's disease large ulceration which is associated with active disease [1] was detected with 100% sensitivity and there were no false positives. Regarding the other barium features, occasionally it was impossible for the radiologist to assess the degree of inflammation in a stricture using barium studies and a range of 99mTc-HMPAO scan scores was seen at the site of these strictures. One stricture gave a negative scan and was assumed to be purely fibrotic which was later confirmed surgically. Of the seven patients with strictures and positive 99mTc-HMPAO scans, 2 patients came to laparotomy, 33 and 54 days later. Biopsy revealed severe active inflammation at the stricture site which was resected in one case and "closed" for steroid treatment in the other. The remaining five patients all responded to steroid treatment alone [16]. In essence, for the patient with small bowel obstructive symptoms, both tests may be necessary and are complementary in directing treatment strategies based on accurate knowledge of the site, extent and activity of disease

Infection in Inflammatory Bowel Disease.

Patients with IBD may develop an intra-abdominal abscess, particularly in Crohn's disease following deep transmural ulceration, Abdominal abscesses are an important cause of post operative morbidity and mortality [5][8], and can present as localised tenderness and fever, or more insidiously without localising signs, resulting in delayed diagnosis [59] and increased mortality. It is therefore crucial to diagnose abscesses as reliably and quickly as possible and ultrasound is usually the first line investigation in most patients because it is rapid and non-invasive [60]. However it has limitations in the post operative patient due to impaired access because of surgical drains and dressings. Moreover, collections cannot always be identified as an abscess rather than serous fluid or haematoma [61].

If the patient has no localising signs, ultrasound has a limited role. In this situation, white cell scanning has been advocated as the investigation of choice [62]. Thakur and Segal first described the use of 111-Indium labelled autologous leucocytes to localise abscesses in dogs [6][3], and then in febrile patients [64]. Their studies using 111-Indium leucocytes showed that intense, focal increasing activity on serial images up to 24 hours was diagnostic of an abscess due to continued recruitment of labelled cells into a confined space; whereas bowel inflammation resulted in decreasing activity with time due to shedding of labelled cells into the bowel lumen and distal transit. Since then, several other authors have confirmed their findings, [65]. In another report [66], 100 consecutive patients were studied using Indium-

111 labelled leucocytes including 34 following surgery, 36 with IBD, 13 with pyrexia of unknown origin (PUO) and 17 with miscellaneous abdominal and pelvic sepsis resulted in a sensitivity of 93% with 100% specificity and in another study of 257 cases over five years with suspected intra-abdominal infection; 97% and 91% respectively [67]. In difficult cases the complementary role of ultrasound, 111-Indium leukocyte scans and CT scanning has been found useful [62].

99m-Technetium -HM-PAO [10] has great potential for the imaging of inflammation. However, non-specific intestinal activity which is particularly prominent after 3 hours 13, resulting in low grade bowel activity at 24hrs, could make the diagnosis of abscesses potentially difficult. As there have been no direct comparisons of these labelling techniques at one, three and twenty four hour time points with same day ultrasound scanning, we compared them all. The established technique of 111-Indium labelled granulocyte scanning was taken to be the gold standard for abscess diagnosis while aspiration was also used when available. A total of 50 adult patients with suspected intra-abdominal abscess were investigated, 25 of whom were known to have IBD. The remaining patients mainly had post-operative fever. IBD patients (particularly Crohn's disease) could present with fever, abdominal pain and a palpable mass. The distinction between bowel wall inflammation and a complicating abscess is particularly important. In Crohn's disease patients, abscesses form spontaneously in 9 - 28% of patients [68]. If left untreated, the abscess may either perforate into a related adherent structure, creating a fistula, or rupture into the peritoneal cavity causing generalised peritonitis. Sixteen of the 21 patients with Crohn's disease presented with a Crohn's mass. All patients were initially investigated with an ultrasound scan. The patients then went on to have white cell scanning on the same day using simultaneous 99m-Tc-HM-PAO labelled mixed white cells and 111-Indium labelled purified granulocytes.

All patients who met the criteria for an abscess on the 111-Indium scan i.e. persistent focal intense uptake at 24 hours also met these criteria on the 99m-Tc-HM-PAO scan resulting in a sensitivity and specificity for intra-abdominal abscess detection using 99m-Tc-HMPAO of 100% (table 2).

Test	Sensitivity	Specificity	Accuracy	Predictive Values	
				+ve	-ve
Ultra Sound	62%	87%	73%	0.73	0.88
99mTc HM-PAO	100%	100%	100%	1.0	1.0

Table 2. *Comparison of ultrasound and 99m-Tc-HM-PAO to 111-Indium scanning.*

Mild colonic activity on 24hr 99m-Tc-HM-PAO images did not interfere with image interpretation at all (figure 6).

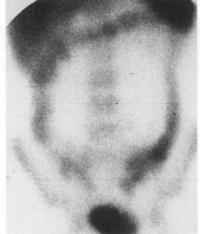

Figure 6 (a) *Initial 99m-Tc-HM-PAO scan showing total Crohn's colitis and terminal ileitis at 1 hour. Prominent bladder activity is shown.*

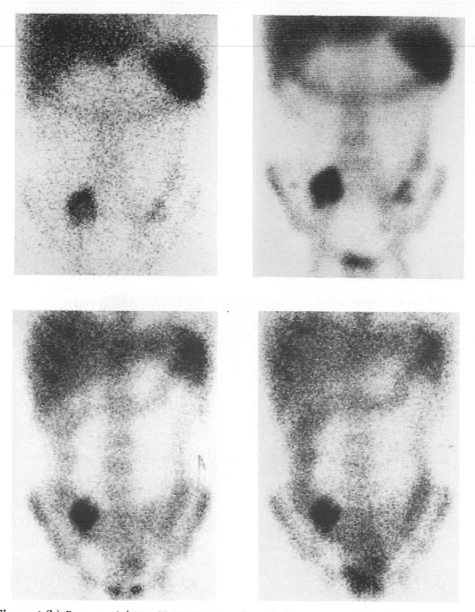

Figure 6 (b) *Repeat serial 99m-Tc-HM-PAO and 111-Indium scans performed 19 days later due to development of a right iliac fossa mass and tenderness showing the appearance of an abscess (bi, and biii are 1 hour and 24 hours 111-Indium scans; bii and iv are 999m-TC-HM-PAO 1 hour and 24 hour scans.*

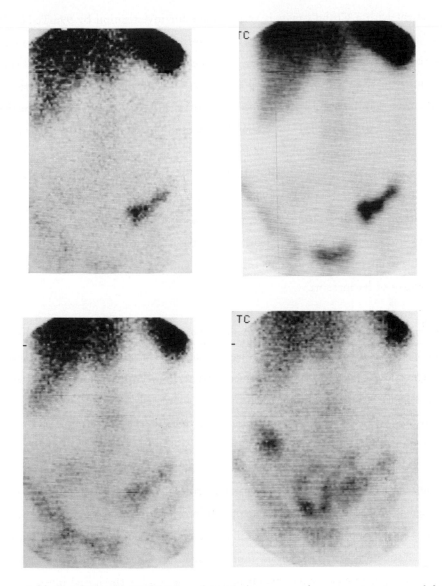

Figure 6 (c) *Serial 99m-Tc-HM-PAO and 111-Indium scans demonstrating intense left iliac fossa activity on early images but loss of activity at 24 hours due to diverticulitis. Note non specific colonic activity in right iliac fossa at 24 hours on 99m-Tc-HM-PAO image which does not cause diagnostic problems.(ci and iii are 1 hour and 24 hour 111-Indium scans; cii and iv are 99m-Tc-HM_PAO 1 hour and 24 hour scans*

The patient with a Crohn's mass is very suitable for investigation by 99mTc-HM-PAO white cell scanning as using this method, abscesses are accurately detected as well as the degree of associated bowel inflammation. Also the typical appearance of small bowel loops at 1 hour with transit into large bowel at 3 hours with no focal uptake, left little doubt that the mass was due to matted inflamed loops of small bowel and in clinical practice no 24 hour scan would be needed [16] as found in the study by Lantto et al [69]. Our findings indicating the usefulness of 99mTc-HM-PAO scanning in intra-abdominal abscess detection confirm a recent retrospective study of 69 patients with suspected abdominal abscesses which demonstrated a sensitivity of 90%, specificity of 91% and accuracy of 91% using this technique; ultrasound was less accurate, with a sensitivity of 74% [69], similar to our own findings. White cell scanning was useful in three patients with fever in whom ultrasound was unable to distinguish haematoma from abscess and negative white cell scans supported the diagnosis of haematoma.

Most importantly, a normal one hour 99m-Tc-HM-PAO scan excludes any inflammation including an abscess, providing a rapid exclusion diagnosis while 1hr 111-Indium scans are not diagnostic and not normally performed. Twenty four hour imaging is essential using both methods. When 111-Indium labelled mixed white cells are used instead of purified granulocytes (as is often the case), the sensitivity for abscess detection is 67% at 4hrs compared to 100% at 24hrs [70]. Colloid subtraction to remove background liver activity is usually recommended to image liver abscesses [71].

CT scanning has an important complementary role in abdominal sepsis [62]. It has the advantage of providing more precise anatomical information and is particularly useful for the investigation of pancreatic sepsis. It can detect collections of fluid with high sensitivity but the distinction between serous fluid, haematoma and abscess may be difficult. Aspiration if possible can solve this dilemma. Ultrasound is the initial investigation of choice due to its rapid availability and simplicity and reported superiority in liver lesions [60]. If this is unhelpful or equivocal then either CT or 99mTc-HMPAO scanning should be performed. If there is still doubt then the third modality should be used. If a chronic low grade infection is suspected then 111-Indium is the investigation of choice.

In conclusion we recommend that 99mTc-HMPAO is the non-invasive investigation of choice for imaging IBD. For complicating abdominal sepsis, ultrasound remains the initial investigation of choice however, particularly in the post - operative patient and if results are equivocal or inconsistent with clinical findings, then the patient should be further investigated with radio labelled white cell scanning or CT scanning [62]. 99mTc-HMPAO imaging is as sensitive and specific as 111-Indium scanning in the diagnosis of intra-abdominal abscess with improved availability, reduced radiation dosage, technical simplicity and in cases of exclusion of an abscess, a rapid result and it is therefore the second line investigation of choice.

Acknowledgements:

I would like to thank Dr Maxwell and Joe Joseph for their supervision of this work and for being part of the G-I imaging team at St. George's hospital who have worked with me on various white cell scanning projects including Jeff Gane, Catherine Lowe, Arash Masoomi and Alan Britten.

References

1. Goldberg HI, Brooke JR. Recent advances in the Radiographic Evaluation of Inflammatory Bowel Disease. Med Clin North Am 1980;64:1059-1081.
2. Watts JMK, de Dombal FT, Goligher JC. Early results of surgery for ulcerative colitis. Br J Surg 1966;53:1005-1014.
3. Metchnikoff E. Immunity in infective diseases. Cambridge: Cambridge University Press, 1905: 175-206.
4. Dancey J, Deubelbeiss K, Harker L, Finch C. Neutrophil kinetics in man. J Clin Invest 1976;58:705-715.
5. Lavender JP, Lowe J, Barker JR, Burn JI, Chaudhri MA. Gallium- 67 citrate scanning in neoplastic and inflammatory lesions. Br J Radiol 1971;44:361-366.
6. Mc Afee J, Thakur M. Survey of radioactive agents for in vitro labelling of phagocytic leucocytes. 1. Soluble agents. J Nucl Med 1976;17:480-7.
7. Keshavarzian A, Price YE, Peters AM, Lavender JP, Wright NA, Hodgson HJ. Specificity of indium-111 granulocyte scanning and faecal excretion measurement in inflammatory bowel disease--an autoradiographic study. Digest Dis Sci 1985;30:1156-60.
8. Zakhireh B, Thakur ML, Malech HL, Cohen MS, Gottschalk A, Root RK. Indium-111-labelled human polymorphonuclear leukocytes: viability, random migration, chemotaxis, bactericidal capacity and ultrastructure. J N Med 1979;20:741-747.
9. Saverymuttu S, Camilleri M, Rees H, Lavender J, Hodgson H, Chadwick V. Indium 111-granulocyte scanning in the assessment of disease extent and disease activity in inflammatory bowel disease. A comparison with colonoscopy, histology, and faecal indium 111-granulocyte excretion. Gastroenterology 1986;90:1121-8.
10. Peters AM, Danpure HJ, Osman S, Hawker RJ, Henderson BL, Hodgson HJ, Kelly JD, Neirinckx RD, Lavender JP. Clinical experience with 99mTc-hexamethyl-propyleneamineoxime for labelling leucocytes and imaging inflammation. Lancet 1986;2:946-9.
11. Neirinckx RD, Canning LR, Piper IM, et al. Tc-99m d,l-HM-PAO: A new radiopharmaceutical for SPECT imaging of regional cerebral blood perfusion. J Nucl Med 1987;28:191- 202.

12. Scholmerich J, Schmidt E, Schumichen C, Billmann P, Schmidt H, Gerok W. Scintigraphic assessment of bowel involvement and disease activity in Crohn's disease using technetium 99m-hexamethyl propylene amine oxine as leukocyte label. Gastroenterology 1988;95:1287-93.

13. Becker W, Schomann E, Fischbach W, Borner W, Gruner KR. Comparison of 99Tcm-HM-PAO and 111In-oxine labelled granulocytes in man: first clinical results. Nucl Med Commun 1988;9:435-47.

14. Shrimpton P, Wall B, Jones D, Fisher E, Hillier M, Kendall G, Harrison R. A national survey of doses to patients undergoing a selection of routine X-ray examinations in English hospitals. National Radiation Protection Board, 1986.

15. Peters AM, Roddie ME, Danpure HJ, Osman S, Zacharopoulos GP, George P, Stuttle AW, Lavender JP. 99Tcm-HM-PAO labelled leucocytes: comparison with 111In-tropolonate labelled granulocytes. Nucl Med Commun 1988;9:449-63.

16. Weldon M. 99mTc-HM-PAO Planar White Cell Scanning. Scand J Gastroenterol 1994;29:36-42.

17. Modigliani R, Mary J Y, Simon J F, et al. Clinical, biological and endoscopic picture of attacks of Crohn's disease; evolution on prednisolone. Gastroenterology 1990;98:811-18.

18. Gibson P, Lichtenstein M, Salehi N, Hebbard G, Andrews J. Value of positive technetium-99m leucocyte scans in predicting intestinal inflammation. Gut 1991;32:1502-7.

19. Lantto EH, Lantto TJ, Vorne M. Fast diagnosis of abdominal infections and inflammations with technetium-99m-HMPAO labeled leukocytes. J Nucl Med 1991;32:2029-34.

20. Papos M, Nagy F, Lang J, Csernay L. Technetium-99m hexamethyl-propylene amine oxime labelled leucocyte scintigraphy in ulcerative colitis and Crohn's disease. Eur J Nucl Med 1993;20:766-9.

21. Vilien M, Nielsen SL, Jorgensen M, Binder V, Hvid JK, Berild D, Kelbaek H. Leucocyte scintigraphy to localize inflammatory activity in ulcerative colitis and Crohn's disease. Scand J Gastroenterol 1992;27:582-6.

22. Sciarretta G, Furno A, Mazzoni M, Basile C, Malaguti P. Technetium-99m hexamethyl propylene amine oxime granulocyte scintigraphy in Crohn's disease: diagnostic and clinical relevance. Gut 1993;34:1364-9.

23. Peters A. Imaging inflammation: current role of labelled autologous leukocytes [editorial]. J Nucl Med 1992;33:65-7.

24. Saverymuttu SH, Maltby P, Batman P, Joseph AE, Maxwell D. False positive localisation of indium-111 granulocytes in colonic carcinoma. Br J Radiol 1986;59:773-7.

25. Becker W, Fischbach W, Weppler M, Mosl B, Jacoby G, Borner W. Radiolabelled granulocytes in inflammatory bowel disease: diagnostic possibilities and clinical indications. Nucl Med Commun 1988;9:693-701.

26. Saptogino A, Becker W, Wolf F. 99mTc-labelled polyclonal human immunoglobulin for localisation of inflammatory sites--early in vitro-results. Nucl Med 1990;29:54-8.

27. Hebbard GS, Salehi N, Gibson PR, Lichtenstein M, Andrews JT. 99Tcm-labelled IgG scanning does not predict the distribution of intestinal inflammation in patients with inflammatory bowel disease. Nucl Med Commun 1992;13:336-41.

28. Joseph K, Hoffken H, Bosslet K, Schorlemmer HU. Imaging of inflammation with granulocytes labelled in vivo. Nucl Med Commun 1988;9:763-9.

29. Locher JT, Seybold K. White blood cell scintigraphy. Problems related to the use of monoclonal antibodies. Prog Clin Biol Res 1990;355:327-36.

30. Boyd SJ, Nour R, Quinn RJ, McKay E, Butler SP. Evaluation of white cell scintigraphy using indium-111 and technetium-99m labelled leucocytes. Eur J Nucl Med 1993;20:201-6.

31. Peters A, Lavender J, Danpure H, Osman S, Saverymuttu S. Tc-99m autologous phagocyte labelling: a new imaging technique for inflammatory bowel. Br Med J 1986;293:450-1.

32. Lennard-Jones JE. Classification of inflammatory bowel disease. Scand J Gastroenterol 1989;24:2-6.

33. Clamp SE, Myren J, Bouchier IAD, Watkinson G, De Dombal FT. Diagnosis of inflammatory

bowel disease: an international multicentre scoring system. Br Med J 1982;284:91-95.

34. Pera A, Bellando P, Caldera D, et al. Colonoscopy in inflammatory bowel disease.Diagnostic accuracy and proposal of an endoscopic score. Gastroenterology 1987;92:181-5.

35. Best W, Becktel J, Singleton J, Kern F. Development of a Crohn's disease activity index. National Co-operative Crohn's disease study. Gastroenterology 1976;70:439-44.

36. Hodgson HJF. Assessment of drug therapy in inflammatory bowel disease. Br J Clin Pharmacol 1982;14:159-70.

37. Camilleri M, Proano M. Advances in the assessment of disease activity in inflammatory bowel disease. [Review]. Mayo Clinic Proc 1989;64:800-7.

38. Bartholomeusz FD, Shearman DJ. Measurement of activity in Crohn's disease. [Review]. J Gastroenterol Hepatol 1989;4:81-94.

39. Hanauer SB. Guidelines for the clinical evaluation of drugs for patients with inflammatory bowel disease. Fed Register 1991;56:519.

40. Modigliani R, Mary Y-J. Groupe d'etudes therapeutiques des affections inflammatoires digestives. Clinical, biological and endoscopic picture of attacks of Crohn's disease. Evolution on prednisolone. Gastroenterology 1990;98:811-818.

41. Jenkins D, Goodall A, Drew K, et al. What is colitis? Statistical approach to distinguishing clinically important change on rectal biopsy specimens. J Clin Pathol 1988;41:72-9.

42. Saverymuttu SH, Peters AM, Crofton ME, Rees H, Lavender JP, Hodgson HJ, Chadwick VS. 111Indium autologous granulocytes in the detection of inflammatory bowel disease. Gut 1985;26:955-60.

43. Carpani de Kaski M, Peters AM, Knight D, Stuttle AW, Lavender JP, Hodgson HJ. Indium-111 whole-body retention: a method for quantification of disease activity in inflammatory bowel disease. J Nucl Med 1992;33:756-62.

44. Spinelli F, Milella M, Sara R, et al. The 99mTc-HMPAO leukocyte scan: an alternative to radiology and endoscopy in evaluating the extent and the activity of inflammatory bowel disease. J Nucl Biol Med 1991;35:82-7.

45. Giaffer MH, Tindale WB, Senior S, Barber DC, Holdsworth CD. Quantification of disease activity in Crohn's disease by computer analysis of Tc-99m hexamethyl propylene amine oxime (HMPAO) labelled leucocyte images. Gut 1993;34:68-74.

46. Stein P, Gray G, Gregory P, Anderson M, Goodwin D, McDougall I. Location and activity of ulcerative and Crohn's colitis by indium-111 leukocyte scan. Gastroenterology. 1983;84:388-93.

47. DeNardo G, Macey D, DeNardo S, Zhang C, Custer T. Quantitative SPECT of uptake of monoclonal antibodies. Sem Nucl Med 1989;19:22-32.

48. Weldon MJ, Masoomi AM, Britten AJ, Gane J, Finlayson CJ, Joseph A, Maxwell JD. Quantification of inflammatory bowel disease using technetium-99m-HMPAO labelled leucocyte Single Photon Emission Computerised Tomography (SPECT). Gut 1995;36:243-250.

49. Truelove S, Witts L. Cortisone in ulcerative colitis: final report on a therapeutic trial. Br Med J 1955;1041-4.

50. Lantto E, Jarvi K, Krekela I, et al. Technetium-99m hexamethyl propylene amine oxine leucocytes in the assessment of disease activity in inflammatory bowel disease. Eur J Nucl Med 1992;19:14-8.

51. Almer S, Franzen L, Peters AM, et al. Do technetium-99m hexamethylpropylene amine oxime-labeled leukocytes truly reflect the mucosal inflammation in patients with ulcerative colitis? Scand J Gastroenterol 1992;27:1031-8.

52. Rosenbusch G, Jansen JB, Reeders JW. Contemporary radiological examination of the small bowel. In: Tytgat GNJ, Reeders JWAJ ed. Diagnostic imaging of the gastrointestinal tract: part 1. London: Bailliere Tindall, 1994: 683-700.

53. Saverymuttu SH, Peters M, Hodgson JH, Chadwick VS, Lavender JP. 111Indium leukocyte scanning in small bowel Crohn's disease. Gastrointest Radiol 1983;8:157-161.

54. Park RH, McKillop JH, Duncan A, MacKenzie JF, Russell RI. Can 111indium autologous mixed

leucocyte scanning accurately assess disease extent and activity in Crohn's disease? Gut 1988;29:821-5.

55. Crama BG, Arndt JW, Pena AS, et al. Value of indium-111 granulocyte scintigraphy in the assessment of Crohn's disease of the small intestine: prospective investigation. Digestion 1988;40:227-36.

56. Froelich JW, Field SA. The role of Indium-111 white blood cells in inflammatory bowel disease. Sem Nucl Med 1988;18:300-307.

57. Kennan N, Hayward M. Tc HMPAO-labelled white cell scintigraphy in Crohn's disease of the small bowel. Clin Radiol 1992;45:331-4.

58. Fry DE, Garrison RN, Heitsch RC, Calhoun K, Polk JHC. Determinants of death in patients with intraabdominal abscess. Surgery 1980;88:517-523.

59. Saverymuttu S, Peters A, Lavender J. Clinical importance of enteric communication with abdominal abscesses. Br Med J 1985;290:23-26.

60. Joseph AE. Imaging of abdominal abscesses [editorial]. Br Med J Clin Res 1985;291:1446-7.

61. Doust BD, Quiroz F, Stewart JM. Ultrasonic distinction of abscesses from other intra abdominal fluid collections. Ultrasound 1977;125:213-217.

62. Knochel JQ, Koehler PR, Lee TG, Welch DM. Diagnosis of abdominal abscesses with computed tomography, ultrasound, and 111In leukocyte scans. Radiology 1980;137:425-32.

63. Thakur ML, Coleman RE, Mayhall CG, Welch MJ. Preparation and evaluation of 111In labelled leukocytes as an abscess imaging agent in dogs. Radiology 1976;119:731-732.

64. Segal A, Thakur M, Arnot R, Lavender J. 111 Indium labelled leucocytes for localisation of abscesses. Lancet 1976;13:1056-1058.

65. Coleman RE, Black RE, Welch DM, Maxwell JG. Indium-111 labeled leukocytes in the evaluation of suspected abdominal abscesses. Am J Surg 1980;139:99-104.

66. Goldman M, Ambrose NS, Drolc Z, Hawker RJ, McCollum C. Indium-111-labelled leucocytes in the diagnosis of abdominal abscess. Br J Surg1987;74:184-6.

67. Baldwin JE, Wraight EP. Indium labelled leucocyte scintigraphy in occult infection: a comparison with ultrasound and computed tomography. Clin Radiol 1990;42:199-202.

68. Steinberg DM, Cooke WT, Alexander-Williams J. Abscess and fistulae in Crohn's disease. Gut 1973;14:865-9.

69. Lantto EH. Leucocytes labelled with 99mTc-HMPAO in the detection of abdominal abscesses. Eur J Surg 1991;157:469-72.

70. Mountford P, Kettle A, O'Doherty M, Coakley A. Comparison of Technetium-99m-HM-PAO leukocytes with indium 111-oxime leukocytes for localising intra abdominal sepsis. J Nucl Med 1989;31:311-315.

71. Datz LF, Luers P, Baker WJ, Christian PE. Improved detection of upper abdominal abscesses by combination of 99mTc sulfur colloid and 111Indium leukocyte scanning. Am J Radiol 1985;144:319-323.

CHAPTER 9

IMAGING ABDOMINAL SEPSIS

D.P.Clarke and J.R.Buscombe

Introduction

Infection within the abdomen is a common clinical problem affecting both patients in the community and in hospital. Infections may vary from mild self limiting gastro-enteritis to multiple life threatening opportunistic infections in the immunocompromised. When diffuse organ system involvement with infection is present there is often a clinical, biochemical or serological indicatorof the underlying source of the infection, for example jaundice and deranged liver function tests in acute hepatitis. Whilst US and CT will show changes compatible with active inflammation and exclude co-existant problems such as gallstones, they have little to add to further management. Similarly simple infections of the genito-urinary and gastro-interstinal tracts are usually diagnosed by clinical and routine bacteriological means, imaging and endoscopy being reserved for difficult cases.

Abdominal abscesses occur in a wide variety of abdominal sites, may involve any organ system and have a number of different causes. When dealing with focal pyogenic and inflammatory change within the abdomen the clinician is hampered by the innaccuracy of clinical and plain radiographic signs: US and CT employ different physical properties of tissue but share an excellent ability to differentiate fluid collections from soft tissue. Increasingly this ability has been used for minimally invasive percutaneous drainageof fluid collections obviating the need for formal surgery. Diagnosing the site and cause for intra-abdominal sepsis using plain radiography has proven both difficult andvery susceptible to observer error [1]. Following the introduction of both ultrsound [US] and computed tomography [CT], the likely applications and benefits of these techniques within the abdomen were soon realised. The trans-axial imaging plane offered by US and CT allow direct visualisation of the anatomical relationships of, and extent of, focal infection within the abdomen. With the advent of helical CT, multiplanar imaging is nowa reality for both techniques. In addition, the speed of helical CT increases the throughput and availability

P. H.Cox and J. R. Buscombe (eds.), The Imaging of Infection and Inflammation, 183–197.
© 1998 *Kluwer Academic Publishers. Printed in the Netherlands.*

and also increases contrast resolution. Helical CT also reduces misregistration artefacts and allows rendering of high quality three dimensional models [2]. This is likely to lead to improved definition and characterisation of abdominal sepsis [3]. Coupled to this have been advances in scintigraphic techniques initially with Gallium-67 Citrate and then with labelled leucocytes [4][5][6]

A number of salient qualities are unique to each technique and will be uninfluenced by current technological innovations. Ultrasound is portable, inexpensive and does not involve ionising radiation, but is highly operator dependent, gives a limited visualisation of the retro peritoneum and does not adequately visualise the spine or paraspinous soft tissues. Computed tomography gives excellent anatomical resolution including bowel interloop areas and the retro peritoneum but is moreexpensive, employs ionising radiation and is susceptible to sub optimal bowel opacification. Nuclear Medicine provides the ability to image the whole abdomen easily and is unaffected by changes in anatomy caused by surgery etc however techniques can be expensive and time consuming. As technological advances render equipment more expensive, limited access will continue to be a problem.

Hepatic Sepsis

Focal hepato-biliary sepsis is readily identifiable on US, 80% of pyogenic abscesses being identified [7], usually in the right lobe. On CT they are sharply demarcated with a characteristic enhancing capsule and a low density centre often containing gas [8] [figure 1]

The identification of bright ecogenic foci on ultrasound suggests gas formation and a recent report [9] emphasises its high incidence in diabetic patients in whom the prognosis is worse. Hepatic abscesses can be simulated by necrotic metastases which can become infected and ultimately surgery, or percutaneous guided drainageprocedures are required to achieve diagnosis and treatment [Fig 2] [10]. The cure rate with this technique is 72.6% for immunocompetent patients compared with 53.1% for immunocompromised individuals with a failure rate of 8.9% [11]. Patients with intra hepatic communication display similar cure rates but require longer duration of drainage [12]. amoebic abscesses appear similar but

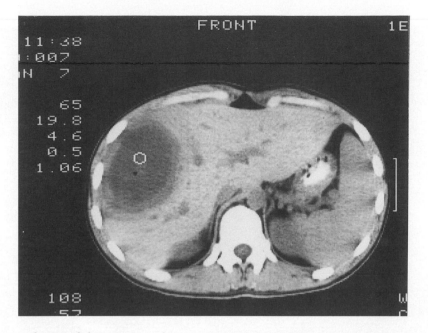

Figure 1. *The CT of this patient with a pyogenic liver abscess demonstrates focal low density with a well defined capsule. There is a tiny pocket of air seen in the centre of the abscess implying a gas-forming organism.*

on US lack rim echoes to suggest a wall [7] and on CT rarely display the septations seen in pyogenic abscesses [8].

Hydatid infection can be diagnosed on US alone provided it produces one of the classical appearances [multi septated cyst, daughter cysts, detached membrane or calcified wall] together with positive serology [13]. Unfortunately other morphological varieties [purely cystic or heterogenous mass] are more common and are nonspecific both on US and CT [8]. Simple hepatic cysts have an incidence of 2.5% [7] but usually have CT and US appearances that allow easy discrimination. Simple hepatic abscesses can be imaged as photopenic areas on a Technetium-99m sulphur colloid study. The sensitivity of this method can be improved by by using single photon emission tomography [SPET]. The use of Gallium-67 Citrate or labelled leucocytes is more problematical as both of these agents have significant uptake into the liver as part of the reticulo endothelial system.

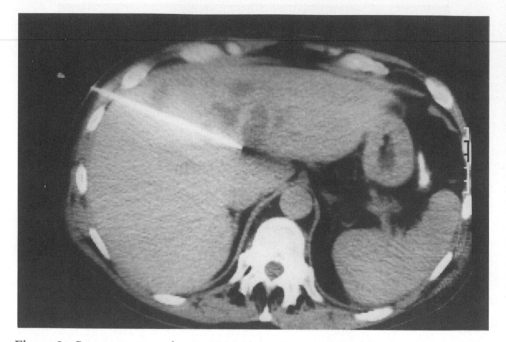

Figure 2. *Percutaneous transhepatic CT guided aspiration of a multiloculated pyogenic abscess centred on the quadrate lobe*

Any uptake into an abscess may be masked by normal liver tissue [14]. Strategies to overcome this include: i] imaging over time so that the abscess shows increasing uptake whilst the liver remains static [fig 3], ii] an additional Technetium-99m colloid scan after imaging of the liver has concluded with substraction techniques used to "remove" normal liver tissue, iii] use of SPET to increase contrast resolution. It should also be possible to provide better localisation of any abnormality within the liver.

Biliary Sepsis.

Biliary sepsis occurs in obstruction and in primary cholangitis. Infection normally occurs in the presence of gallstones. Ultrasound findings rely on the presence of stones in the gallbladder or the common bile duct and bile duct enlargement [greater than 8mm], sensitivities reported are between 19and 80% [15][16].

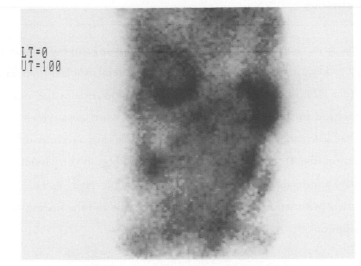

Figure 3. *48 hour gallium-67 citrate study showing a hepatic abscess in the right lobe with ring of increased activity around a photopaenic necrotic centre.*

Computed tomography canal so accurately define biliary dilation and identify stones. Overall CT is less operator and interpreter dependent than US and this may be the reason for the lesser variability reported in sensitivity of CDB stone detection for CT [45-90%] than that of US [17]. That approximately 30% ofpatients with ductal stones do not display dilated ducts [15] remains a diagnostic problem for both US and CT. Hepatobiliary scintigraphy using second or third generation Technetium-99m labelled iminodiacetic acids [IDA's] have a useful role in the diagnosis of acute cholecystis and also bile duct obstruction. In acute cholecystis the swelling of the cystic duct prevents passage of activity into the gallbladder therefore non visualisation of the gall bladder within 4 hours of injection of the Tc-99m IDA has a sensitivity of >95% in a series of studies totalling 1000 patients [18]. This process can be quickened by the use of morphine at 0.1mg/kg which is given at the end of one hour. If the gallbladder is not visualised in the next thirty minutes then thestudy isconsidered positive [19]. Due to the relatively poorer availability of both on on call nuclear medicine and CT, ultrasound remains the screening procedure for putative biliary sepsis providing a quick, non invasive examination which also allows assessment of gall bladder inflammation.

Sub-phrenic infection.

The sub-phrenic space is often implicated in patients following surgery or after liver sepsis. Infections may produce localising symptoms such as ipsilateral shoulder tip pain but canalso be without either localising symptoms or signs. Ultrasound remains the ideal method for identifying infection in the sub-phrenic space however when negative either gallium-67 citrate or labelled leucocytes are indicated. If these are used then a technetium-99m sulphur colloid subtraction [Fig 4] though SPET may be of help [14]. If the patient has localising signs or a positive scintigraphy study then CT is indicated. Normally however, scintigraphy is used in a patient with sepsis but without localising signs and the finding of sub-phrenic sepsis is serendipitous.

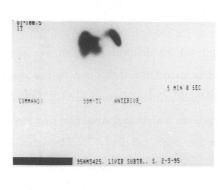

Figure 4. *Patient with a sub-phrenic abscess. The top image is a technetium-99m sulphur colloid scan performed 1 hour after injection. This image is then subtracted from the 48 hour gallium-67 citrate image (middle image). The resulting subtraction image (bottom row) clearly demonstrates subphrenic accumulation of gallium-67 citrate not visible on the planar image.*

Splenic infection.

Splenic enlargement in systemic infection is a common finding and is easily assessed with

US and can also be seen in gallium-67 citrate and labelled leucocyte imaging. Abscess isless common and may be secondary to haematologous spread, infarction or immunodeficiency. Ultrasound guided puncture is an effective diagnostic and therapeutic option. With gallium-67 citrate imaging splenic uptake is often less than in the liver and focal uptake can be seen. With labelled leucocytes particularly those labelled with technetium-99m hexamethylpropylene amine oxine [HMPAO] labelled splenic uptake is often significant. therefore acolloid subtraction technique is useful if a splenic abscess is suspected.

Infections of the gastrointestinal tract.

Barium contrast planar radiography has classically been used to evaluate bowel disease but the cross sectional component of both US and CT allow visualisation of the bowel wall and, to some extent, its component structures. Acute inflammatory oedema and chronic inflammatory thickening and scarring can be identified on US and employing endoscopic high frequency sonography allows distinction of individual layers of the bowel wall. Another important feature of bowel ultrasound is the realtime evaluation of peristalsis. However it may be difficult to differentiate between changes due to scarring from old disease and new acute changes. Ultrasound can also be of use in the differentiation of adynamic ileus [e.g. in peritonitis] from obstruction. Whilst scintigraphic techniques such as labelled leucocytes can be sensitive in the identification of bowel infection it may be impossible to differentiate between this and a bowel inflamed due to inflammatory bowel disease.

Further problems arise in the use of different scintigraphic techniques. Gallium-7 citrate has normal excretion into the bowel at the level of the caecum. Therefore by 24 hours activity of gallium-67 in the colon is non-specific. The normal strategy used to determine if colonic gallium-67 activity is indeed pathological is to perform sequential scans over a 48 or 72hour period. This can be very time consuming and useless in a patient with ileus. With indium-111 labelled leucocytes images can be performed up to 24 hours post injection and all bowel activity considered pathological. Technetium-99m HMPAO labelled leukocytes havesome activity in normal bowel from about 3.5 hours post injection, therefore it is recommendedthat with this agent abdominal imaging beperformed at 1and 3 hours post injection [20][Fig 5.].

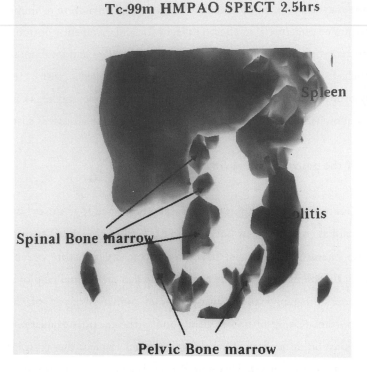

Figure 5. *Three dimensional volume rendered image of the abdomen of a patient with an infective colitis performed at 2.5 hours. Normal structures such as the bone marrow, liver and spleen are noted as well as the site of colitis in the decending colon.*

A complication of inflammatory bowel disease is a Chrohn's abscess. This may be visualised CT, US or labelled leukocytes. CT and US are more useful in those patients who have no previous surgery and in whom the anatomy is normal. In patients who are post surgical then labelled leucocytes may be superior [21]. Because of its normal bowel activity galliu-67 citrate is not recommended. Indium-111 labelled leukocytes are probably the agent of choice as good quality images can be performed at 24 hours post injection. Images of the bowel can alsobe performed at 24 hours post injection of technetium-99m HMPAO leukocytes. However the 1 and 3 hour images are used to look for bowel infection. A late 24 hour image is also performed, bowel activity is ignored as normal but any new focal areas of uptake are considered to be due to a Crohn's abscess [22].

Pseudomembranous colitis is an infectious colitis that occurs most frequently as a complication of antibiotic therapy. Diffuse and segmental involvement of thelarge bowel is described, the wall displaying a shaggy contour and mural thickening; anaccordion pattern has been shown to be highly suggestive of pseudomembranous colitis and consists of contrast trapped between thickened haustral folds which are aligned parallel [23]. The paucity of associated pericolonic inflammation in this disorder helps to differentiate it from other forms of colitis [24].

Diverticulitis and its complications are identified with high sensitivity by CT which has recently been confirmed to be superior to the contrast enema [25]. The diagnosis of appendicitis remains a challenging clinical problem the frequently atypical clinical presentation giving rise to a laparotomy rate of around 20%. Computed tomography and graded compression US are the modalities of choice in evaluation. Recently it hasbeen suggested that CT is superior to US, as it was found to have a higher sensitivity, negative predictive value and accuracy although specificity and positive predictive values were comparable. Scintigraphic techniques described in identifying acute appendicitis include gallium-67 citrate and labelled leukocytes [26]. However the sinsitivity of these techniques rarely exceeds 80% as there is often little inflammation in early disease.

There is a problem in that imaging of gallium is difficult in the abdomen before 24 hours. This means that if the clinician waits for the result of the gallium-67 citrate scan they may belooking at the effect of a post rupture appendicular abscess!. Labelled leukocyte scanning may also be of utility in this condition and the scanning can be completed in 4-6 hours post request [27]. It has also been shown that using technetium-99n antigranulocyte antibodies, imaging at one hour post injection has the same sensitivity of 90-95% aslater imaging in acute appendicitis [28]. Therefore such a method which can give a rapid answer may become more widely used in those patients presenting with suspected acute appendicitis.

Intra-peritoneal sepsis.

Intraperitoneal infection can be more difficult to detect clinically than visceral sepsis.

Clearly the history can be crucial [recent surgery or trauma] and familiarity with the peritoneal reflections and retroperitoneal anatomy promotes the most complete and accurate interpretation of imaging studies. Abscesses without prior surgery or trauma areless common but may arise from appendicitis, diverticulisis or pelvic inflammatory disease [1] [29]. Opinions differ as to the most sensitive and appropriate imaging technique but in practice the modality employed is often determined by the experience and preferenceof the operator. Ultrasound is highly effective in the right upper quadrant and pelvis but in the left subphrenic space, thelesser sac and intra-abdominal interloop area overlying bowel gas may render CT superior to US [30].

Percutaneous catheter drainage of intra-abdominal abscesses has become a widely accepted radiological practice [Fig 6].

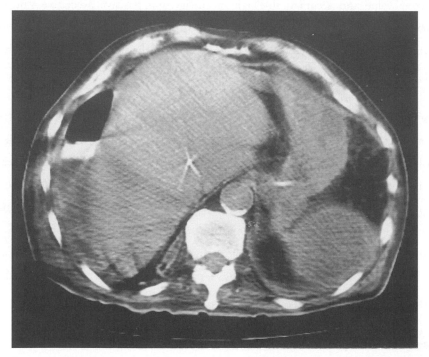

Figure 6a.

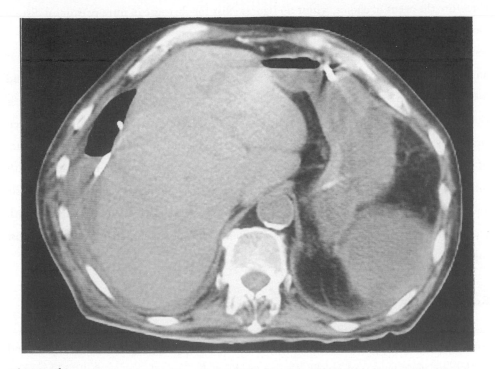

Figure 6b.

Figure 6. *CT Scans of a patient with ulcerative colitis six weeks following sub-total colectomy. The rectally administered contrast [fashioning an ileal reservoir was planned] has leaked into the right sub-phrenic abscess [6a] which was effectively drained percutaneously under CT control [6b].*

Needle aspiration alone is recommended for small collections [less than 3cm] [31]. Recent US applications in the diagnosis of pelvic inflammatory disease may prove useful in the future; demonstration of low resistance blood flow in tubo-ovarian infectious complex by trans-vaginal sonography in out patients as a sensitive and specific means of early detection [33]. The place of nuclear medicine is in those patients in whom initial ultrasound or CT has been non-contributary or in those patients where it is known that the anatomy and interpretation of anatomical data alone may be difficult. Due to the previously mentioned non-specific bowel uptake of gallium-67 citrate is not appropriate, labelled leukocytes is therefore the agent of choice, whilst no figures exist for their use in intra-peritoneal disease alone series of patients including those with including those with intra-peritoneal have a sensitivity of 76% and a specificity of 83% [34]. Focal infection can be easily identified as an area of increasing labelled leukocyte accumulation and this is normally seen in the 1 and 3-4 hour labelled leukocyte images [20]. The role of focal uptake of labelled leukocytes is then to allow aspiration of pus under ultrasound or CT control. Similar results have been suggested with technetium-99m labelled anti-granulocyte antibodies but only a small series of patients have been reported [35]. General peritonitis gives a very different pattern with diffuse activity seen over the whole of the centre of the abdomen. Changes can be subtle and may be difficult to identify, late images in this case may be useful though with technetium-99m HMPAO labelled leukocytes any bowel uptake after four hours post injection should not be considered pathological.

Retroperitoneal infection.

Acute renal infection is normally identified clinically by the prescence of local pain and tenderness with fever and pyuria. In uncomplicated acute infections of the kidney, no radiological workup in the adult is indicated. Radiological evaluation is indicated only in the severely ill, immunocompromised individual and patients who fail to responf to antibiotics [36]. If imaging is required the ideal study of choice for a hospitalised patient with suspected renal infection is CT as it is more sensitive for demonstrating the presence of acute renal pathology, localising thesite of infection [intra-renal, perinephric, pararenal etc]. In uncomplicated acute infections of thekidney, however, ultrasound will provide useful information by examining for obstruction, stonesand congenital abnormalities.

Scintigraphy using gallium-67 citrate has been applied to thesepatients [37][38] and good results can be obtained. For example multiple sites of uptake throughout both kidneys with pulmonary uptake has been seen in renal tuberculosis. Labelled leukocytes can also be used however there has been some suggestion that human immunoglobulin labelled with indium-111 may be superior to indium-111 labelled leukocytes [39]. Technetium-99m labelled pharmaceuticals are of less use in renal disease because of the renal excretion of pertechnetate or other technetium-99m labelled metabolites of either labelled leukocytes or antigranulocyte antibodies. An alternative strategy would be to look for defects in the technetium-99m dimercatosuccinic acid [DMSA] scan. Acute infection can show as a small area of swollen kidney, some area of poorly defined renal outline or as a clear defect [40]. Its main use however is in the assessment of scarring post infection. The use of technetium-99m DMSA is therefore not considered part of the standard investigation od patients with suspected renal infection.

Pyogenic infection in the other post retro-peritoneal sites such as the pancreas or thepsoas muscles is readily seen on both US and CT and are amenable to percutaneous aspiration. Scintigraphic techniques are not primarily osed to confirm infection at these sites though they may have a useful role to play in determining if any infection has been successfully treated.

Conclusion.

In many respects the diagnostic and therapeutic functions of US and CT complement each other in the search for intra-abdominal infection. Thus although CT can often produce more detailed information and more reliably define the anatomical extent of sepsis, US lends itself to immediate bedside examination which can be frequently repeated if clinical doubt remains. Scintigraphic techniques within the abdomen are limited to labelled leukocytes, due to the non-specific bowel uptake of gallium-67 citrate. A labelled leukocyte study should be considered in the following cases: 1] patients with a high index of suspicion for abdominal infection but no localising symptoms or signs, 2] those patients in whom initial ultrasound or CT has been unhelpful, 3] those patients with abnormal anatomy where the interpretation of either ultrasound or CT may be difficult. It must also be recognised that these studies are not competitive but complimentary and as such a fusion of the knowledge obtained from at least two of these modalities is often essential. Definitive diagnosis, when necessary, can be made by guided needle aspiration od suspicious collections or by surgical exploration.

References

1. Connell TR, Stephens DH, Carlson HC, et al. Upper abdominal abscess: A continuing and deadly problem. Am J Roentgenol 1980.134.759-765.
2. Zeman RK, Fox SH, Silverman PM, et al. Helical [spiral] CT of the abdomen. Am J Roentgenol 1993.160.719-725.
3. Rubin GD, Silverman G. Helical [spiral] CT of the retroperitoneum. Radiol Clin N Am 1995.33.903-930.
4. Staab EB, McCartney WH. Role of gallium-67 in inflammatory disease. Sem Nucl Med 1978.8.219-234.
5. Thakur ML, Lavender JP, Arnot RN, et al. Indium-111 labelled autologous leukocytes in man. J Nucl Med 1977.18.1014-1021.
6. Peters AM. The utility of [99m] Technetium HMPAO leukocytes for imaging infection. Sem Nucl Med 1994.242.110-127.
7. Marn CS, Bree RL, Silver TM. Ultrasonography of liver: Technique and focal and diffuse disease. Radiol Clin N Am 1991.29.1151-1167.
8. Vassilades VG, Bree RL, Korobkin M. Focal and diffuse benign hepatic disease: correlative imaging. Sem Ultrasound CT MRI 1992.13.313-335.
9. Yang CC, Chen CY, Lin XZ, et al. Pyogenic liver abscess in Taiwan: emphasis on gas forming liver abscess in diabetics. Am J Gastroenterol 1993.88.1911-1915.
10. Pitt HA. Surgical management of hepatic abscesses. World J Surg 1990.14.498-504.
11. Lambiaise RE, Deyoe I, Cronan JJ, et al. Percutaneous drainage of 335 consecutive abscesses: results of primary drainage with one year follow up. Radiology 1992.184.167-179.
12. Lambiaise RE, Deyeo I, Cronan JJ, et al. Percutaneous drainage of hepatic abscesses: comparison of results in abscesses with and without intrahepatic biliary communication. Am J Roentgenol 1991.1209-1212.
13. Gharbi HA, Hassine W, Brauner MW, et al. Ultrasound examination of the hydatid liver. Radiology 1981.139.459-463.
14. Mountford J, Coakley AJ. Radiolabelled agents for the localisation of infection. In: Nuclear Medicine in clinical diagnosis and therapy. Vol1. Ed: Murray I.P.C. and Ell P.J.1995 Churchill Livingstone, London. pp129-140.
15. Laing FC, Jeffrey RB. Choledocholithiasis and cystic duct obstruction. Difficult ultrasound diagnosis. Radiology 1983.146.471-474.
16. Baron RL. CT diagnosis of choledocholithiasis. Sem Ultrasound CT MRI.1987.8.85-102.
17. Laing FC, Jeffrey RB, Wing VW. Improved visualisation of Choledocholithiasis by sonography. Radiology 1986.110.39-42.
18. Freitis JE. Cholescintigraphy in acute and chronic cholecystitis. Sem Nucl Med 1982.12.18-26.
19. Fink-Bennett D. Augmented cholescintigraphy: its role in detecting acute and chronic disorders of the hepatobiliary tree. Sem Nucl Med 1991.21.128-139.
20. Mountford PJ, Kettle AG, O'Doherty MJ, et al. Comparison of technetiu-99m -HMPAO leukocytes and indium-111-oxine leukocytes for localising intra-abdominal sepsis. J Nucl Med 1990.31.311-315.
21. Mcdougal IR,Goodwin DA,Silverman P, et al. Comparison of indium-111 labelled white cell scans and ultrasonography in detection of intra-abdominal abscess. Clin Nucl Med 1980.4.558-559.
22. Wheeler JD, Slack N, Duncan A. The diagnosis of intra-abdominal abscesses in patients with severe Crohns disease. Q J Med 1992.82.159-167.

23. Fishman EK, Kavaru M, Jones B, et al. Pseudomembranous colitis; CT evaluation of 26 cases. Radiology 1991.180.57-60.

24. Merine D, Fishman EK, Jones B. Pseudomembranous colitis: CT evaluation. J Comp Ass Tomog 1987.11.1017-1020.

25. Jacobs JE, Birnbaum BA. CT of inflammatory disease of the colon. Sem Ultrasound CT MRI 1995.16.91-101.

26. Navarro DA, Weber PM, Hodgson JH, et al. Indium -111 leukocyte imaging in appendicitis. Am J Roentgenol 1987.148.733-736.

27. Childs J, Buscombe J, Marshall D, et al. Using audit and algorithms in the scintigraphic imaging of infection. J Nucl Med Tech 1995.23.262-266.

28. Overbeck B, Briel B, Hotze A, et al. 99m-Tc-antigranulocyte antibodies [BW250/183] in the detection of appendicitis. Nucl Med 1992.31.24-28.

29. Field TC, Pickleman J. Intra-abdominal abscess unassociated with prior operation. Arch Surg 1985.120.821-824.

30. Jasinski RW, Glazer GM, Francis IR, et al. CT and US in abscess detection at specific anatomic sites. Comp Radiol 1987.11.41-47.

31. Casola G, van Sonnenberg E, D'Agostino HB, et al. Percutaneous drainage of tubo ovarian abscess. Radiology 1992.182.399-402.

32. Tinkanen H, Kujansuu E. Doppler ultrasound findings in tubo ovarian infectious complex. J Clin Ultrasound 1993.21.175-178.

33. Cacciatore B, Leminen A, Ingman-Friberg S, et al. Transvaginal sonographic findings in ambulatory patients with suspected pelvic inflammatory disease. Obst Gynecol 1992.80.912-916.

34. Weldon MJ, Joseph AEA, Saverymutu SH, et al. Comparison of Technetium-99m-HMPAO labelled leukocyte and indium-111 labelled granulocytes and ultrasound in the diagnosis of intra-abdominal abscess. Gut 1995.37.557-564 35.

35. Becker W, Sapintogino A, Wolf F. Diagnostic accuracy of a late technetium-99m antigranulocyte antibody scan in inflammatory or infectious diseases. J Nucl Med 1991.32.1002.

36. Goldman SM, Fishman EK. Upper urinary tract infection: The current role of CT, ultrasound and MRI. Sem Ultrasound CT MRI 1991.12.3350360.

37. Mendez G, Morillo G, Alanso M, et al. Gallium-67 radionuclide image in acute pyelonephritis. Am J Roentgenol 1980.134.17-22.

38. Kao CH, Wang SJ, Lioa SQ, et al. Usefulness of gallium-7 citrate scans in patients with disseminated tuberculosis and comparison with chest X rays. J Nucl Med 1993.34.1918-1921.

39. Oyen WJG, Claessens RAMJ, van der Meer JWM, et al. Detection of subacute infectious foci with indium-111 labelled autologous leukocytes and indium-111 labelled human non-specific immunoglobulin G: a prospective study. J Nucl Med 1991.32.1854-1860.

40. Majd M, Rushton HG. Renal cortical scintigraphy in the diagnosis of acute pyelonephritis. Sem Nucl Med 1992.22.98-111.

CHAPTER 10

BONE AND SOFT TISSUE

Wolfgang Becker

Introduction

Acute osteomyelitis is clinically suspected in patients with fever, pain, swelling[tumor] and redness as well as warmth, leukocytosis and increased erythrocyte sedimentation rate. The clinical diagnosis of acute osteomyelitis in certain anatomical areas [spine, thigh] with a thick soft tissue surrounding and the diagnosis of chronic osteomyelitits may be difficult. Anyway the early diagnosis and specific diagnosis in posttraumatic patients and diabetic foot patients is essential for a good recovery of the patient without any general or local complication. The clinical problem [i.e. postoperatively] is the differentiation of a normal postoperative irritation or a beginning infection or an infected hematoma. In all these conditions is a need for an infect specific method to help the clinican to answer his questions i.e. - antibiotics: yes or no or operation yes or no.

Morphologic based examinations are not able to give an early diagnosis of infection, because structural changes, osteolytic lesions, dystrophia and periostal reactions can be seen 2 - 3 weeks after the beginning of infection. Magnetic resonance imaging, computed tomography and sonography play no role in the postoperative situation, due to their lack of infect specificity. Nuclear Medicine has developped different unspecific and infect specific radiopharmaceuticals for the diagnosis of osteomyelitis and accompagning soft tissue infections.

This review aims to summarize and report all clinical available data on sensitivity and specificity of the different radiopharmaceuticals, which are commercially widely available, in different clinical situations.

P. H.Cox and J. R. Buscombe (eds.), The Imaging of Infection and Inflammation, 199-217.
© 1998 Kluwer Academic Publishers. Printed in the Netherlands.

Tc-99m bone scintigraphy

Due to the hyperemia with increased blood flow, the increased blood pool and mineralization around and within the focus of osteomyelitis, the three phase bone scan should be the first examination, especially in patients with hematogenous osteomyelitis. So in children with suspected osteomyelitis, this is the only necessary examination. This high sensitivity is well known [1,2] and has recently been published again [3]. In this study the diagnostic accuracy has been calculated to be only 20%, due to a lot of possible other reasons for a positive bone scan. Due to its lack of specificity a three phase bone scan only rules out osteomyelitis being negative [4]. If an increased mineralization is suspected due to an immediate preceeding surgery or trauma [4 to 6 months] or in patients with diabetic foot ulcers the bone scan is of limited value and can be omitted. It has been shown that for assessment of the response to therapy Tc-99m-bone scan is not helpful, because after 6 months the scans still showed a positive uptake [5].

Tc-99m-Nanocolloids

In certain respects, Tc-99m-nanocolloid scintigraphy offers important advantage over other infect specific nuclear medicine procedures. It requires considerably shorter investigation times [30 - 60 min] and is easy to handle because it involves neither time consuming preparation of leucocytes in special facilities or technical expertise. In other aspects Tc-99m-nanocolloids are unspecifically taken up in infectious sides, whereas labelled leucocytes specifically. With this tracer alone a few studies have evaluated its diagnostic accuracy and results indicate values similar to these of In-111-leucocyte scintigraphy [Tab.1].

Author	Tc-99m-nanocolloids			Tc-99m/In-111 white cells		
	sensitivity	specificity	accuracy	sensitivity	specificity	accuracy
Abramovic	95%	77%	Ga-67	93%	55%	
Flivik	93%	73%	78%	75%	82%	80%
Streule	87%	93%		81%	93%	
Vorne	59%	100%		97%	100%	

Table.1 *Survey of sensitivity specificity and accuracy of Tc-99m labelled nanocolloids in patients with osteomyelitis.*

The difference between In-111-white cell imaging and Tc-99m-nanocolloids in the cases of chronic osteomyelititis in which Tc-99m nanocolloids correctly identified infection where In-111-leucocytes showed false negative results, may be explained by the different distribution mechanism of the two tracers. The labelled leucocytes are only chemotactically attracted to places with acute inflammation, in chronic osteomyelitits they are hardly involved. On the other hand nanometer-sized colloids continue to find their way into the extravascular space independant of the duration and etiology of the inflammatory process. In certain clinical situations where an additional bone scan is necessary both examinations can be performed within of one day [i.e. 100-150 MBq Tc-99-m-nanocolloids and 2h later 750-900 MBq Tc-99m-phosphates]. It has to be stressed that in the diagnosis of soft tissue diseases no good diagnostic accuracy is available [50%] with Tc-99m-nanocolloids and should therefore not be performed [10].

In-111-labelled autologous leucocytes

Acutely, an infection is characterized by a neutrophilic response. So positive accumulations in patients studied with autologous leucocytes are described as infections. But one has always to keep in mind, that this technique is highly specific for a leucocyte infiltration in a pathologic process, but not specific for a single disease.

So a lot of "false" positive accumulations in different diseases were described [11], especially if we focus on the bone and joints. So positive images may occur after marrow aspiration or at bone graft donor sites [12], faint uptakes are described in some healing fractures. But in nearly all healing noninfected fractures the scans are negative [13]. Well-formed heteroptopic periarticular bone formations [myositis ossificans] in the early stages and neoplasmas [14].

The acute response subsides over time and is replaced by a monocyte/macrophage response, but only 2% to 8% of the reinjected cell suspension are monocytes. So the evidence of a pathologic reaction in these more chronic infections is only the cold lesion in a leucocyte study.

The main indication for leucocyte scintigraphy in bone and soft tissue diseases, prostethic infection excluded, which are discussed in another chapter of this book, are long bone osteomyelitis in children and adult, mostly occuring after traumatic lesions, osteomyelitis of the spine and osteomyelitis in the periphery of the bone, which often occurs in diabetic patients and their diabetic foot.

Patients with the suspicion of long bone osteomyelitis, especially in its acute phase, are referred to leucocyte scintigraphy mostly after traumatic lesions or surgery. Leucocyte scintigraphy in these patients is helpful, because bone scintigraphy is positive anyway and gives only sometimes additional information. There are only a few studies available, which exclusively examine these population of patients. McCarthy et al [15] found excellent results with an overall sensitivity of 97% and a specificty of 82% in bioptically proven osteomyelitis. All these patients had a highly suspicion of osteomyelitis and were probably acute and obviously all of the patients had long bone osteomyelitits in areas without normal bone marrow. Different results are published in patients with chronic osteomyelitis [16]. In a study in patients with infections of different durations the sensitivity of labelled leucocytes for acute infections [less than 2 weeks] was 100% but fell to 73% in more chronic infections [greater than 2 weeks duration] [17]. Another study of the effect of chronicity on the sensitivity of labelled leucocyte imaging did not show any significant difference between acute [sensitivity: 90%] and chronic infection [sensitivity: 86%] [16]. It is generally accepted, that an antibiotic therapy does not influence the sensitivity of leucocyte scintigraphy, if at the time of the study there is still an indication to perform the test [i.e.: pain, swelling and so on] [18].

As a general rule the activity of the disease[chronic, acute] and the localization of the infection is very important. Acute infections can be detected with a sensitivity of about 90%, independent from its localization in the periphery , appendicular or in the central skeleton. Chronic infections have also a high sensitivity in the periphery of about 90%, but decreases to about 50% in the spine[19]. Some authors believe , that this is mainly due to the low spatial resolution of In-111 infiltration in the infectious foci.   The prevalence of osteomyelitis in diabetic foot ulcers is unknown. Early diagnosis of this infection is critical, as prompt antibiotic treatment decreases the rate of amputation.   In patients with diabetes often osteoarthropathy occurs. This is due to the changes in the sensory nerves and subsequent trauma to the affected areas. Besides diabetes also peripheral nerve damage, spinal cord injury , birth defects, tumors , infections and syphilis can be responsible. Osteomyelitis can be difficult to evaluate using conventional   methods when there are superimposed bony changes form the neutrotrophic osteoarthropathy. Radiographically, neutropathic bone has mixed sclerotic and lytic changes, which makes differentiation from osteomyelitis difficult. The three phase bone scan increased the specificity for osteomyelitis, but it loses specificity, when the suspected osteomyelitis is superimposed upon neurotrophic osteoarthropathy or other conditions which cause increased bone turnover. Tab. 2 gives an overview on diagnostic studies with In-111-labelled leukocytes, which come all to the same conclusion.

Author	sensitivity	specificity	accuracy	positive predictive values	negative
Diabetic foot and foot ulcers:					
Keenan	100%	78%	87%		
Maurer	75%	89%		75%	89%
Newman	89%	69%	82%		
Schauwecker	100%	83%			
Osteomyelitis of the Spine:					
Georgi	0%	100%			
Palestro	39%	98%	76%	92%	73%
Other forms and localisation of osteomyelitis:					
Al Sheikh	80%	75%			
Georgi	93%	85%			
McCarthy	97%		82%		92%

Table 2. *Survey of data on the diagnostic accuracy of In-111 labelled white blood cell scans in patients with different forms of osteomyelitis.*

Leukocyte scans are highly sensitive for diagnosing osteomyelitis in diabetic foot ulcers and may so be useful for monitoring the efficacy of antibiotic treatment[22]. Given the low sensitivities of all other noninvasive clinical and laboratory characteristics, an accurate imaging technique is crucial. The leucocyte scan proved to be the most sensitive imaging test with a lower specificity of 69%[22]. The superiority of the leukocyte scan as compared with the bone scan may reflect both the high incidence of false positive bone scans seen in patients with Charcot joints as well as the leucocyte scan's theoretical ability to detect the presence of white blood cells in bone earlier than the bone scan can detect increased osteoblastic activity. Problems arise in the differentiation of soft tissue infection and soft tissue and bone infection. This problem is always present . Only left or right sided images may help in an accurate differentiation. Newman et al [22] recommend to treat all patients with ulcers and exposed bone with antibiotics, because they nearly all have osteomyelitis. But all the patients with ulcer and non exposed bone should undergo leukocyte scintigraphy. After these results of infection in the periphery of the bone the low sensitivity of leukocyte scintigraphy, regarding a positive uptake in a lesion, will be discussed. TAB. 2 gives the results of studies, where osteomyelitis presenting as a zone of photopenia in the spine. Similar observations have been published in further publications [27,28,29,30,31,32,33]. It has been postulated that this photopenia results from occlusion of the microcirculation of the involved bone resulting in acute inflammation and necrosis [34]. Infection induced death of reticuloendothelial cells that normally accumulate labeled leukocytes may also play a role [35]. Another hypothesis might be the high intravertebral pressure in a focus of spine osteomyelitis, which does not allow an uptake of further cells within of the image time of 24h. This phenomenon especially can be seen in patients with significantly longer duration of symptoms [> 3 weeks] [fig.1] than in individuals presenting with in-creased activity on leukocyte images [36].

So the appearance of vertebral osteomyeltis on leukocyte imaging may be dependant, at least in part, on the pathophysiology of the disease itself and the predominant cellular immune response at the time of imaging. Skeletal photopenia on leukocyte images is nonspecific and has also been observed in tumors, previous radiation therapy, fractures, avascular necrosis, myelofibrosis, Paget's diseas and fibrous displasia [27,28,29,30,31,32,33, 37, 38, 39, 40, 41]. Therefore In-111-leukocyte imaging is non diagnostic for osteomyelitis. Most of the detailed studies on different localizations of infection are performed with In-111 as a label. Indium-111 has some disadvantages due to its availability, its high energy and longer physical half-life, which leads to a high radiation exposure to the patients. Due to this fact In-111 should be substituted with Tc-99m-HMPAO, if possible, which is readily available and has best physical characteristics [42].

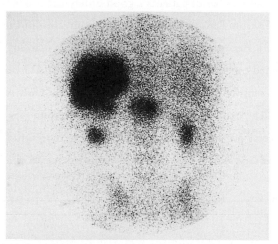

Figure 1. *Patient undergoing chronic hemodialysis with only a two day history of fever,leukocytosis and back pain. The indium-111 oxine leucoscan in a posterior projection clearly demonstrates leukocytic infiltration in the first lumbal spine and in both shrunken kidneys asasign of primary nephritis with metastatic osteomyelitis of the spine. X ray of the spine turned positive on day 13 of the first symptoms.*

Tc-99m-HMPAO-leucocytes

But the given studies with Tc-99m-HMPAO labelled leukocytes in patients with osteomyelitis are less, but principally the mechanism of uptake in the lesion should be comparable to In-111-labelled cells. One disadvantage might be, that Tc-99m as a label has a significant elution out of the cells, which leads to a lower contrast [target/background] in the late scans 24 h after reinjection of the cells [43]. Another difference to In-111 compounds is, that Tc-99m-HMPAO selectively labels the leukocytes, the amount of labelled monocytes is significantly lower [44]. In the largest series of reported examinations, the best indications for HMPAO leukocyte scintigraphy was found to be patients with implants [not only hip replacements but also fixation plates....] or chronic osteomyelitis [45] especially when clinical, biological and radiological signs do not show coincidence of infection. False positives may occur in patients with hematoma or unusual medullary sites. In these cases Tc-99m-sulfur colloid scans are helpful for the differentiation. Also chronic ulcers and perforating ulcers in diabetic patients have been examined and demonstrated in a small number of patients a good differentiation between bone infection and subcutaneous infection. Data in patients with osteomyelitis of the spine are until now not available [TAB.3]. According to these published data, it seems justified to examine patients with suspected osteomyelitis only with Tc-99m HMPAO labelled leukocytes and to expect the same sensitivity and specificity with Tc-99m-HMPAO cells as has been published for In-111 oxin leukocytes in detail. Despite its higher resolution, Tc-99m-HMPAO seems not to be more accurate because more often imaging of chronic osteomyelitis is necessary, where late scans are required due to the limited granulocyte turnover.

Author	sensitivity	specificity	accuracy	positive predictive	negative values
Devillers	100%	100%		100%	100%
(Implants	95%	90%		88%	96%)
El Esper	83%	100%			
Morgas	81%	93%			
Roddie	100%	93%			
Vorne	80%	100%			
Winker	97%	85%			

Table 3. *Survey on data on the accuracy of Tc-99m-HMPAO labelled white blood cells in patients with osteomyelitis*

Tc-99m labelled antigranulocyte antibodies.

The advantage of immunoscintigraphy over autologous leukocyte techniques in the imaging of infection is the simplicity of its use compared with techniques that require the isolation of autologous white blood cells. In bone infection the sensitivity of antigranulocyte scintigraphy in 106 patients was calculated to be 69% for the hips, 79% for the thighs, 85% for the knees and 100% for the lower leg and ankle [51]. The sensitivity decreased from the periphery of the bone to the central parts. This may be due to the physiological uptake of the antibody in the bone marrow containing parts of the bone, where the normal uptake of the antibody does not allow normal bone marrow to be distinguished from small infectious foci. Other hypotheses discuss increased pressure in the vertebral bodies in cases of infection, which prevents labelled white cells or antibodies from penetrating [fig.2].

Encouraging results have been reported in patients with diabetic foot. Images were done within of 4 to 6 hours after injection. The 24h scans showed no additional information. The authors report only one negative scan in a 9 month course of chronic osteomyelitis. False positive results were seen in cellulitis. Although bone scan alone is not helpful in these patients, because bone abnormalities are nearly always present and are more extensive than leukocyte scan involvement, it is recommended to perform an additional bone scan for anatomical reference and for best localization of a lesion.

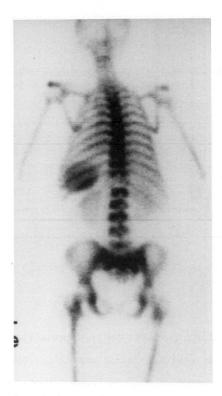

Figure 2. *45 year old female with three weeks history of back pain and cold spot in the Tc-99m antigranulocyte antibody scan 4h p.i. in a histologically proven osteomyelitis of the spine.*

Ga-67-citrate

Ga-67 entails high radiation exposure, is not readily available and has unfavourable physical characteristics for gammacamera imaging . These features combined with the availability of Tc-99m-labelled radiopharmaceuticals for imaging infections, limit the use of Ga-67 citrate to certain indications[42]: One of these is chronic osteomyelitis of the spine. In the periphery of the bone it has been proven, that in patients with chronic osteomyelitis radiographs are of no value in determing activity, since they did not change[54],whereas Ga-67 citrate scans are more useful than Tc-99m bone scans for assessing response to therapy. But autologous leukocyte scintigraphy has comparable sensitivity and specificity[4] and should be preferred.

Author	sensitivity	specificity	accuracy	positive predictive	negative values
Osteomyelitis:					
Hotse	89%	64%	75%	67%	88%
Reuland	57%	75%	67%	67%	67%
hip	69%	93%	81%		
thigh	79%	86%	81%		
knee	85%	83%	84%		
Tibia	100%	100%	100%		
Diabetic Foot:					
Dominguez-Gadea 93%		69%	79%	67%	94%

Table 4. *Survey on data on the accuracy of Tc-99m-antigranulocyte antibody scintigraphy in patients with osteomyelitis*

Autologous leukocytes in the spine always offer photopenia. The data are limited for Ga-67 citrate, but it may be superior to all other radiopharmaceuticals in osteomyelitis, although it is less specific and shows tumors as well and is also a bone seeking agent   which picks up osteoblastic activity. The specificity of Ga-67 and Tc-99m bone scan interpretation can be increased , if special attention is paid to the congruency or relative intensitiy of tracer uptake in the lesion by comparison with that in the rest of the skeleton. In cases of more intense Ga-67 uptake than Tc-99m phosphonate uptake infection is highly probable [fig.3].

Tc-99m-In-111- human unspecific immunoglobulin [HIG]

In-111-HIG is not commercially available, but a lot of studies have been published on this
  radiopharmaceutical. In a first study in patients with bone and joint diseases a 100%
accuracy resulted [55]. Other groups showed excellent sensitivities and specificities in more
than 100 patients[50] Low grade staphylococcus infections were missed in only two
patients. The results of these studies also emphasize that In-111 IgG   accumulate both in
infection and in sterile inflammatory processes such as hematomas,   synovitis and recent
fractures[57].

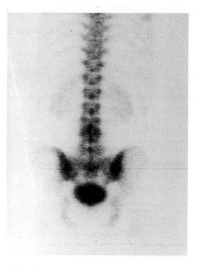
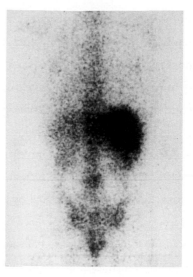

Fig.3a   Fig.3b

Figure 3. *35 year old man with osteomyelitis of the spine and positive bone scan and
comparable uptake in Ga-67 citrate scan in the 3rd/4th vertebra of the spine, which is
indicative for osteomyelitis.*

	Sensitivity	specificity
Oyen	97%	95%
Diabetic foot		
Oyen	86%	84%

Table 5. *Survey on data with In-111 HIG for imaging osteomyelitis and diabetic foot.*

In a group of diabetic foot patients with suspected complications of the foot, In-111 IgG scintigraphy was useful in evaluating the presence or abscence of osteomyelitis at gangrenous or ulcerative lesions [58]. As expected, the conventional bone scan was most sensitive for detecting pedal osteomyelitis, but it was particularly nonspecific in this group of patients. In contrast, In-111-IgG scintigraphy detected 6 of 7 proven osteomyelitis foci, and osteomyelitis was correctly ruled out in 16 of 19 suspected sites.   In a group of 17 patients suspected of having osteomyelitis, the performance of Tc-99m- IgG and Tc-99m BW 250/183 was compared with a final diagnosis established by surgery, histology, and bacteriology. In peripherally located osteomyelitis both agents showed similar and good results. However, in centrally localized osteomyelitis, the performance of the two agents was very difficult because injection of the labeled   polyclonal IgG resulted in 'hot 'lesions, whereas the administration of the mouse   monoclonal showed'cold'lesions[59].

Tc-99m-human unspecific immunoglobulin in arthritis

For the assessment of disease activity in patients with rheumatoid arthritis rheumatologists use subjective variables to quantify arthritis activity. Tc-99m human unspecific immunoglobulin proved to be a reliable marker of disease activity [60]. The mechanism of immuno non-specific IgG accumulation at the site of inflammation is still unclear. Exsudation of plasmaprotein throug a leaking capillary bed, binding to bacteria, specific trapping of IgG by Fc-receptors located in inflammatory cells have been postulated. In comparison with inactive disease the mean joint uptake of Tc-99m HIG with active disease was significantly higher [60] [fig.4].

Also in patients with erosions the joint uptake was significantly higher. Bone scintigraphy
showed no significant difference between both groups. The same is true for patients with
osteoarthritis in comparison to rheumatoid arthritis . Image scores for Tc-99m-IgG joint
scintigraphy correlated highly with scores for joint swelling and C-reactive protein leeds,
weakly with pain scores and not with radiographic scores of joint destruction. So Tc-99m
IgG joint scintigraphy with images 4 h p.i. provide an objective test to detect synovitis
and measure the activity of the disease. In patients with knee joint disease the comparison
of Tc-99m HIG before and 14 days after injection of 20mg triamcinolone resulted in a
decreased arthritis activity measured clinically and histologically. This decrease was paralled
in all patients except one, by a lower uptake of Tc-99m IgG after the injection when
compared to the uptake prior to treatment [61]. These results demonstrate that Tc-99m IgG
joint scintigraphy may provide an objective test to detect synovitis and measure the activity
of the disease.

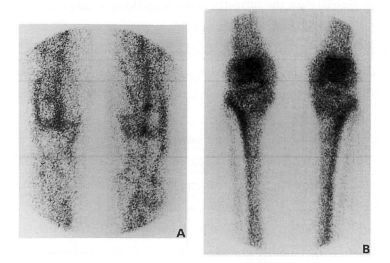

Figure 4. *Patient with rheumatoid arthritis and active disease in the knee joints. [a] Tc-99m
human immunoglobulin scintigraphy clearly demonstrates inflammation of the synovia of both
knees, whereas [b] bone scintigraphy [2h p.i.] only showed increased metabolism of the osseous
structures of the knee as a sign of a chronic process, which does not allow to prove active disease.
Only blood pool [5-10min.p.i.] imaging can give this information.*

Future aspects

Recently the results obtained using Tc-99m Fab-fragments in patients with osteomyelitis have been published [62]. The authors compared the diagnostic accuracy with the accuracy of white blood cell imaging and found a sensitivity, specificity and diagnostic accuracy of 88%,75% and 80% for the fragment and 86%, 78% and 81% for the white blood cell imaging. The new technique was much easier because it employs a one-vial kit which is ready to use 5 min after technetium labelling. It showed the same diagnostic accuracy , but all the clinical information was already provided by the scans obtained 1h p.i. Another advantage over other antibodies was the negligible HAMA response rate. However , as yet this new technique is not routinely available.

Non of the discussed methods is able to answer the surgeon's most important question in a patinet who has clinical signs of inflammation or infection after surgery, namely whether such signs are indicative for infection or merely inflammation.   While inflammation only requires conservative treatment, infection needs further surgical intervention. Nevertheless, the currently available methods do allow some opportunities of differentiation, e.g. if the uptake of a radiopharmaceutical around a knee prostheses is intensive but homogenous, it is probably indicative of inflammation while if it is more focal it is likely to present infection. As a general rule, good interpretation of scans is feasible when they are considered in conjunction with all the available anamnestic and clinical data.

Certain specific steps that have been taken towards the detection of bacterial contamination are worthy of mention. Goldenberg et al. injected Tc-99m-Fab--fragments directed against Pneumocystis carinii and were able to identify patients infected with the microrganism[see this book]. It is therefore possible that rapid diagnosis and localization of other infectious lesions may be feasible using organism-specific, radiolabelled monoclonal antibodies. Another approach is the use of labelled antibiotics, which can be specifically metabolized by different microorganism. The best method is the use of a broad-spectrum antibiotic, as has been achieved with the Tc-99m-labelling of a quinolone called 'infecton'by Bomanji et al [63]. These authors found that imaging of infection was possible, but , more interestingly, scans turned positive before white cell scanning showed any uptake. This may represent a good approach for differential   diagnosis of infection and inflammation.

Nuclear medicine, with its different approaches, images pathophysiology and pathobiochemistry. The available new techniques, especially within immunology and molecular biology, are yielding new insights into the cascade of infection and inflammation. We now understand that via cytokines, especially interleukins, endothelial cells become activated after a chemotactic signal and granulocytes are able to interfere with the expressed molecules, such as E-selectin, before they leave the circulation. The use of In-111-labelled E-selectin fragments is an exciting new method for imaging the expression of E-selectin and to have an epitope on the vascular surface, which allows specific images to be acquired whitout the need of an antibody to pass the vessel wall[64]. However the labelling of interleukin-1 and interleukin-2 is also possible and provides specific signals from infectious and autoimmune diseases [65,66]. The value of these new techniques is the possibility of using peptides in infection. A major problem in the imaging of infection is the fact that nearly every radiopharmaceutical works, because the increased capillary permeability allows radiopharmaceuticals to emigrate from the circulation. For most techniques this yields a high sensitivity but no useful specificity. Small peptides also leave the circulation rapidly, but if they do not specifically bind to their receptor at the focus, they may leave the focus within of a given time. The rapid targeting together with rapid clearance from the focus promise to yield high sensitivity and, more importantly, high specificity in the detection of infection. Since the first report of the chemoattractant properies of small N-formyl peptides[67], these compounds have attracted increasing attention[68]. The results of Fischman et al [69] demonstrate the localization of radiolabelled chemotactic peptide analogs at focal sites of infection in experimental models of deep-thigh infection at sufficient concentrations to permit external imaging soon after intravenous administration. Further improvements of such peptides analogs are, however, required before they can be administered to humans. Future aims for peptide imaging of infection are labelling of a small fraction of the available receptor with a high concentration of radioactivity labelling of the peptide with Tc-99m and achievement of a reduced biological activity, e.g. with antagonists or partial antagonists [69].

References:

1. Lisbona R, Rosenthall L. Observations on the sequential use of Tc-99m phosphonate complex and Ga-67 imaging in osteomyelitis, cellulitis, and septic arthritis. Radiology 1977; 123; 123-9.
2. Rosenthal L, Lisbona R, Hernandez M, Hadjipavlou A. Tc-99m-PP and Ga-67 imaging following insertion of orthopedic devices. Radiology 1979; 133; 717-21 .
3. Becker W, Bair J, Behr Th, et al. Detection of soft-tissue infections and osteomyelitis using a technetium-99m-labelled anti-granulocyte monoclonal antibody fragment. J Nucl Med 1994; 35; 1436-43.
4. Al-Sheikh W, Sfakianakis GN, Mnaymneh W, et al. Subacute and chronic bone infections: diagnosis using In-111, Ga-67 and Tc-99m-MDP bone scintigraphy and radiography Radiology 1985; 155; 501-6 .
5. Alazraki N, Fierer J, Resnick D. Chronic osteomyelitis: Monitoring by Tc-99m-phosphate and Ga-67-citrate Am J Radiol 1985; 145; 767-71.
6. Abramovic J, Rubinstein M. Tc-99m-Nanocolloids: an alternative approach to diagnosis of inflammatory lesions of bones and joints Eur J Nucl Med 1988, 24; 244.
7. Flivik K, Sloth M, Rydholm U, Herrlin K, Lidgren L. Technetium-99m nanocolloid scintigraphy in orthopedic infections: a comparison with Indium-111-labeled leukocytes. J Nucl Med 1993; 34; 1646-50.
8. Streule K, deSchrijver M, Fridrich R. Tc-99m-labelled HSA nanocolloid versus In-111-oxine labelled granulocytes in detecting skeletal septic processes. Nucl Med Commun 1988; 9; 59-67.
9. Vorne M, Lantto S, Paakkinen S, Salo S, Soini I. Clinical comparison of Tc-99m-HMPAO labelled leukocytes and Tc-99m-nanocolloid in the detection of inflammation. Acta Radiol 1989; 30; 633-7 .
10. Wheeler JG, Slack NF, Duncan A, Palmer M, Harvey RF. Tc-99m-nanocolloids in inflammatory bowel disease. Nucl Med Commun 1990; 11; 127-33.
11. McAfee JG, Samin A. In-111-labeled leukocytes: a review of problems in image interpretation. Radiology 155; 1985; 221-9.
12. Propst-Proctor SL, Dillingham MF, McDougall IR, et al. The white blood cell scan in orthopedics. Clin Orthop 169; 1982; 157-65.
13. Mead LP, Scott AC, Bondurant FJ, Browner BD. Indium-111 leukocyte scanning and fracture healing. J Orthop Trauma 4; 1990; 81-4.
14. Schmidt KG, Rasmussen JW, Wedebye IM, Frederiksen PB, Pedersen NT. Accumulation of Indium-111-labeled granulocytes in malignant tumors J Nucl Med 29;1988; 479-84.
15. McCarthy K, Velchik MG, Alavi A, Mandell GA, Esterhai JL, Golf S. Indium-111 labeled white blood cells in the detection of osteomyelitis complicated by a preexistin condition. J Nucl Med 29; 1988; 1015-21.
16. Datz F, Thorne D. Effect of chronicity of infection on the sensitivity of the In-111-WBC scan. Am J Roentgenol 147; 1986; 809-12.
17. Sfakianakis GN, Al-Sheik W, Heal A, et al. Comparisons of scintigraphy with In-111 leukocytes and Ga-67 in the diagnosis of occult sepsis. J Nucl Med 23; 1982; 618-26.
18. Datz FL. The current status of radionuclide infection imaging in: Freeman LM. Nuclear Medicine Annual 1991 Raven Press, Ltd. New York 1993 47-76.
19. Schauwecker DS, Burt RW, Park HM et al. In-111 white blood cell sensitivity depends on the location of the osteomyelitis. Radiology 165; 1987; 72.
20. Keenan AM, Tindel NL, Alavi A. Diagnosis of pedal osteomyelitis in diabetic patients using current scintigraphic techniques. Arch Intern Med 1989; 149; 2262-6.
21. Maurer AH, Millmond SH, Knight LC, et al. Infection in diabetic osteoarthropathy: use of indium-labelled leukocytes for diagnosis. Radiology 1986; 161; 221-5.
22. Newman LG, Waller J, Palestro CJ, et al. Unsuspected osteomyelitis in diabetic foot ulcers. JAMA 1991; 266; 1246-51.

23. Schauwecker DS, Park HM, Burt RW, Mock BH, Wellman HN. Combined bone scintigraphy and indium-111 leukocytes scans in neutropathic foot disease. J Nucl Med 1988; 29; 1651-5.

24. Georgi P, Kaps HP, Sinn HJ. Leukozytenszintigraphie bei entzndlichen Prozessen der Wirbelsule. Radiologie 1985;25; 324-8.

25. Palestro CJ, Kim CK, Swyer AJ, Vallabhajosula S, Goldsmith SJ. Radionuclide diagnosis of vertebral osteomyelitis: indium-111 leukocyte and Tc-99m-methylene diphosphonate bone scintigraphy. J Nucl Med 1991; 33; 1861-5.

26. McCarthy K, Velchik MG, Alavi A, Mandell A, Esterhai JL, Goll S. Indium-111 labeled white blood cells in the detection of osteomyelitis complicated by a pre-existing condition. J Nucl Med 1988; 29; 1015-21.

27. Schauwecker DS. Osteomyelitis: diagnosis with In-111-labeled leukocytes. Radiology 171; 1989; 141-6.

28. Mok YP, Carney WH, Fernandez-Ulloa M. Skeletal photopenic lesions in In-111-WBC imaging. J Nucl Med 25; 1984; 1322-6.

29. Brown ML, Hauser MF, Aznarez A, Fitzgerald RH. Indium-111-leukocyte imaging: the skeletal photopenic lesion. Clin Nucl Med 11; 1985; 611-3.

30. Datz FL, Thorne DA. Cause and significance of cold bone defects on indium-111-labeled leukocyte imaging. J Nucl Med 28; 1987; 820-3.

31. Wukich DK, Van Dam B, Abreu SH. Preoperative indium-labelled white blood cell scintigraphy in suspected osteomyelitis of thc axial skeleton. Spine 13; 1988; 1168-70.

32. Whalen JL, Brown ML, McCleod R, Fitzgerald RH. Limitations of indium-leukocyte imaging for the diagnosis of spine infections. Spine 16; 1991; 193-7.

33. Eisenberg B, Power JE, Alavi A. Cold defects in In-111-labeled leukocyte imaging of osteomyelitis in the axial skeleton. Clin Nucl Med 16; 1991; 103-6 .

34. McCarthy K, Velchik MG, Alavi A, Mandell GA, Esterhai JL, Goll S. Indium-111 labelled white blood cells in the detection of osteomyelitis complicated by a pre-existing condition. J Nucl Med 29; 1988; 1015-21.

35. Wukich DK, Abreu SH, Callaghan JJ, et al. Diagnosis of infection by preoperative scintigraphy with indium-labeled leukocytes. J Bone Joint Surg [A] 69; 1987, 1353-60.

36. Palestro CJ, Kim CK, Swyer AJ, Vallabhajosula S, Goldsmith S. Radionuclide diagnosis of vertebral osteomyelitis: Indium-111 leukocyte and technetium-99m-methylene diphosphonate bone scintigraphy. J Nucl Med 32; 1991;1861-5.

37. Coleman RE, Welch D. Possible pitfalls with clinical imaging of indium-111 leukocytes: concise communication. J Nucl Med 21; 1980; 122-5.

38. Borin BF, Abghari R, Sarkissian A. Skeletal photopenic appearance of Paget`s disease with indium-111 white blood cell imaging. Clin Med Nucl 12; 1987; 783-4.

39. Dunn EK, Vaquer RA, Strashun MA. Paget`s disease: a cause of photopenic skeletal defect in indium-111 wbc scintigraphy. J Nucl Med 29; 1988; 561-3.

40. Palestro CJ, Swyer AJ, Kim CK, Vega A, Goldsmith SJ. Appearance of Paget`s disease on In-111-leukocyte images. J Nucl Med 30; 1989; 755.

41. Swyer AJ, Palestro CJ, Kim CK, Goldsmith SJ. Appearance of fibrous dysplasia on In-111-labeled leukocyte scintigraphy. Clin Nucl Med 16; 1991; 133-5.

42. Becker W. The contribution of nuclear medicine to the patient with infection Eur J Nucl Med 22; 1995;1195-211.

43. Becker W, Schomann E, Fischbach W, Brner W, Gruner KR. Comparison of Tc-99mHMPAO and In-111 oxine labelled granulocytes in man: first clinical results. Nucl Med Commun 9; 1988; 435-47.

44. Peters AM, Danpure HJ, Osman S, et al. Clinical experience with Tc-99m hexamethylpropylene amine oxime for labelling leukocytes and imaging inflammation. Lancet 2; 1986; 946-9.

45. Devillers A, Moisan A, Jean S, Arvieux C, Bourguet P. Technetium-99m hexamethylpropylene amine oxime leukocyte scintigraphy for the diagnosis of bone and joint infections: a retrospective study in 116 patients. Eur J Nucl Med 1995; 22;302-7.

46. El Esper I, Dacquet V, Paillard J, Bascoulergue G, Tahon MM, Fonroget J. Tc-99m-HMPAO labelled leukocyte scintigraphy in suspected chronic osteomyelitis related to an orthopaedic device: clinical usefulness. Nucl Med Commun 1992; 13; 799-805.

47. Moragas M, Lomena F, Herranz R. et al. Tc-99m-HMPAO leukocyte scintigraphy in the diagnosis of bone infection. Nucl Med Commun 12; 1991; 417-27.

48. Roddie ME, Peters AM, Danpure HJ, et al. Inflammation: imaging with Tc-99m-HMPAO-labeled leukocytes. Radiology 1988; 166; 767-72.

49. Vorne M, Soini I, Lantto T, Paakkinen S. Technetium -99m HMPAO labelled leukocytes in the detection of inflammatory lesions: comparison with Ga-67 citrate. J Nucl Med 30; 1989; 1332-6.

50. Winker KH, Reuland P, Weller S, Feine U. Infektionsdiagnostik in der Chirurgie des Bewegungsapparates mit der Tc-99m-HMPAO-Leukozytenszintigraphie Langenbecks. Arch Chir 374; 1989; 200-7.

51. Reuland P, Winker KH, Heuchert T, Ruck P, Mller-Schauenburg W, Weller S, Feine U. Detection of infection in postoperative orthopedic patients with Tc-99m labeled monoclonal antibodies against granulocytes. J Nucl Med 32; 1991; 526-31.

52. Hotze A, Briele B, Overbeck B, et al. Tc-99m-labelled antigranulocyte antibodies in suspected bone infection. J Nucl Med 1992; 33; 526-31.

53. Dominguez-Gadea I, Martin-Curto LM, de la Calle H, Crespo A. Diabetic foot infections: scintigraphic evaluation with Tc-99m-labelled anti-granulocyte antibodies. Nucl Med Commun 1993; 14; 212-8.

54. Alazraki N, Fierer J, Resnik D. Chronic osteomyelitis: monitoring by Tc-99m-phosphonates and Ga-67 citrate imaging. Am J Roentgenol 145; 1985; 767-71.

55. Fishman AJ, Rubin RH, Khaw BA, et al. Detection of acute inflammation with In-111 labeled non-specific polyclonal IgG. Sem Nucl Med 18; 335-44; 1988.

56. Oyen WJG, van Horn JR, Claessens RAMJ, Sloof TJJH, van der Meer JWM, Corstens FHM. Diagnosis of bone joint and joint prosthesis infections with In-111-labelled specific human immunoglobulin G scintigraphy. Radiology 182; 195-9;1992.

57. Oyen WJG, Claessens RAMJ, van Horn JR, van der Meer JWM, Corstens FHM. Scintigraphic detection of bone and joint infections with indium 111 labeled nonspecific polyclonal human immunoglobulin G. J Nucl Med 31; 403-12; 1991.

58. Oyen WJG, Netten PM, Lemmens AM, et al. Evaluation of infectious diabetic foot complications with indium-111 labeled human unspecific immunoglobulin G. J Nucl Med 33; 1330-6; 1992.

59. Sciuk J, Brandau W, Vollet B, et al Comparison of Tc-99m polyclonal human immunoglobulin and Tc-99m monoclonal antibodies for imaging chronic osteomyelitis. Eur J Nucl Med 18; 401-7; 1991.

60. de Bois MAW, Arndt JW, van der Velde EA, et al. Tc-99m human immunoglobulin scintigraphy-a reliable method to detect joint activity in rheumatoid arthritis. J Rheumatol 19;1371-6; 1992.

61. de Bois MHW, Arndt JW, Tak PP, et al. Tc-99m labelled polyclonal human immunoglobulin G scintigraphy before and after intraarticular knee injection of triamcinolone hexacetonide in patients with rheumatoid arthritis. Nucl Med Commun 14; 883-7; 1993.

62. Becker W, Bair J, Behr T, et al. Detection of soft tissue infections and osteomyelitis using a technetium-99m-labeled antigranulocyte monoclonal antibody fragment. J Nucl Med 35; 1436-43; 1994.

63. Bomanji J, Solanki KK, Britton K, Siraj Q, Small M. Imaging infection with Tc-99m-radiolabeled `infecton`. Eur J Nucl Med 20; 834; 1993.

64. Keelaan ETM, Harrison AA, Chapman PT, Binns RM, Peters AM, Haskard DO. Imaging vascular endothelial activation: an approach using radiolabeled monoclonal antibodies against the endothelial cell adhesion molecul E-selectin. J Nucl Med 35;276-81; 1994.

65. Signore A, Parman A, Pozilli P, Andreani D, Beverley PCL. Detection of activated lymphocytes in endocrine pancreas of BB/W rats by injection of I-123-interleukin -2: an early sign of type-1 diabetes Lancet II; 537-41; 1987.
66. Van der Laken, Boerman OC, Oyen WJG, et al. Recombinant human interleukin-1: potential agent to image infectious foci. Eur J Nucl Med 21; 790; 1994.
67. Schiffmann E, Corcoran BA, Wahl SM. Formylmethionyl peptides as chemoattractants for leukocytes. Proc Natl Acad Sci USA 72; 1059-62; 1972.
68. Becker EJ. The formylpeptide receptor of the neutrophil: a search and conserve operation Am J Pathol 129; 16-24; 1987.
69. Fischman AJ, Babich JW, Rubin RH. Infection imaging with technetium-99m-labelled chemotactic peptide analogs. Sem Nucl Med 24; 154-68; 1994.

CHAPTER 11

IMAGING BACTERIAL INFECTION WITH A RADIOLABELLED ANTIBIOTIC

Ravi Kashyap, Sobhan Vinjamuri, Anne V Hall, Satya S Das, Kishore K Solanki, and Keith E Britton.

Introduction

The bio-physiological basis of nuclear medicine imaging is related to the disease process and it has been further developed - this time the target is bacteria and the disease state is infection. It is often than an inflammation may be due to bacterial infection. Conditions like osteomyelitis or endocarditis where long term antibiotic therapy would be appropriate require that the specific presence of a bacterial infection is demonstrated as the cause of inflammation. The available radiopharmaceuticals: Ga-67 citrate, Tc-99m or In-111 human immune globulin, Tc-99m antigranulocyte antibodies or binding peptides or Tc-99m/In-111 labelled leucocytes offer little help to provide this specific information. To address this issue, a search was pursued for an agent which would bind to living bacteria and that can be radiolabelled. This has resulted in development of Tc-99m Infection by Solanki et al [1].

Tc-99m Infection is based on a synthetic broad spectrum antibiotic Ciprofloxallin which is a 4-fluoroquinolone. The method of radiopharmaceutical preparation is simple and does not involve any handling of blood products. Its evaluation was undertaken in an Ethics and Administration of Radioactive Substance Advisors Committee approved study to look at its stability, biodistribution, clinical utility and a comparison with radiolabelled white cell imaging in randomly selected patients with a site of known or suspected infection.

The results shown that the preparation is stable both in vitro and in vivo. It biodistributes from blood pool to the site of bacterial infection besides showing some concentration in liver and kidneys. Unlike the radiolabelled WBC it does not show any significant uptake in bone marrow thus facilitating evaluation of regions like an infected vertebra.
The main route of excretion is through kidneys. The suggested imaging time is one and four hours post administration of the radiotracer. The infected focus is seen to concentrate this agent by one hour and the uptake increases with time at later imaging. It has been

P. H.Cox and J. R. Buscombe (eds.), The Imaging of Infection and Inflammation, 219-227.
© 1998 *Kluwer Academic Publishers. Printed in the Netherlands.*

evaluated in skeletal, abdominal, endocardial, soft tissue and skin infection with the results that are better in sensitivity, specificity and accuracy as compared to the Tc-99m labelled white blood cells imaging. It has been observed in our preliminary experience that effective antibiotic therapy prior to imaging leads to negative results. This pathophysiological basis of imaging bacterial infection with Tc-99m Infection provides an easy, safe and effective method for detecting active bacterial infection.

Infection Approach

Basic Principles

For localization of an infectious process a nuclear medicine procedure with high sensitivity in all areas of the body is required. In order to obtain a high sensitivity in bacteria infection imaging it is theoretically most appropriate to choose an agent with properties to target a wide spectrum of pathogenic bacteria. Antibiotics are known to be effective agents against bacterial infection by their bacteriostatic or bactericidal action. To achieve this, it has to be made sure in their selection, that they would be able to target active bacteria anywhere in the body.

Ciprofloxacin is active against both gram positive and gram negative bacteria and meets this requirement. It is particularly active against salmonella, shigella, campylobacter, neisseria and pseudomonas. It is also active against chlamydia and some mycobacteria. On intravenous administration, it has extensive tissue penetration and is metabolised in the liver before excretion through the renal pathway [2,3]. In vitro studies have shown that the antibacterial action of ciprofloxacin results from binding to and inhibition of bacterial DNA gyrase [4].

Technetium-99m is most widely used tracer in nuclear medicine practice because of its universal availability and ideal physical characteristics. Most of the technetium based radiopharmaceuticals contain the nuclide in a reduced form and in general most Tc-99m complexes are prepared by reduction of pertechnetate with the inorganic reducing agent stannous ions in presence of a complexing agent. In presence of excess of stannous and chelating agents Tc-99m chelations follows a first order kinetics. Solanki et al [1] noted that the efficacy of ciprofloxacin is impaired by the presence of iron due to its chelating properties and therefore postulated that such a compound would bind Technetium-99m.

The resulted in development of Tc-99m Infecton - a radiopharmaceutical based on the 4 fluoroquinolone, ciprofloxacin.

Uptake Mechanism

Most radiopharmaceuticals used in nuclear medicine's imaging of infection target somewhere in the cascade of inflammatory reaction, irrespective of the causative agent. In a clinically evident bacterial infection site, the presence of live bacteria is almost certain. Ciprofloxacin is taken up and bound specifically by living bacteria, inactivating the DNA gyrase which is present in most bacteria [4]. There are also reports that ciprofloxacin acts as a biological response modifier to the regulative pathway of several cytokines [5]. What specific effect is relevant when the tracer dose of ciprofloxacin is combined with Tc-99m is still unclear. However in vitro evaluation has shown that Tc-99m Infecton is taken up and bound by variety of live bacteria including Pseudomonas aeruginosa, Escherichia coli and Staphylococcus aureus. No binding is seen with dead bacteria. It is also taken up by bacterial abscesses but not by sterile abscesses in experimental studies in the New Zealand white rabbit.

Preparation

Tc-99m Infecton is prepared by standard mixing method or by a kit method. In the first approach 2mg of ciprofloxacin, 400 micrograms of formamidine sulphonic acid and 1000 MBq of sodium pertechnetate solution is put in a sterile nitrogen filled vial. Here formamidine sulphonic acid acts as a non-metallic reducing agent. This mixture is boiled at 100°C for 10 minutes. The preparation as this stage has mean radiochemical purity of 55 ± 8%. It is then passed through a sterile sephadex DAE81 column attached to a 0.5 micron filter to sterilise the solution and remove the free Technetium-99m. The resultant radiopharmaceutical preparation has 95% radiochemical purity with about 3% free Tc-99m and is radiochemically stable over 8 hours [1,6]. During the filtration a loss of 6% of the activity takes place.

The new two phase kit method of preparation is simple, takes less time and requires no boiling of the constituents. It has been technically difficult to achieve due to the sensitivity of the reaction method and the insolubility of 4-fluroquinolones. This two phase preparation kit has been tested in vitro and in vivo showing similar characteristics of the original method. In vitro the binding to pseudomonas aeruginosa of 17.9% was achieved compared with 19.3% for the standard mixing method. The initial in vivo results on patients also have been very encouraging [7]. Although this method resulted in relatively higher mean free pertechnetate value of 12 ± 8% in the preparation, the convenience and simplicity of procedure with almost similar results makes it the method of choice for formulation of Tc-99m Infecton.

Imaging Protocols

There is no specific preparation and no need for dietary restriction prior to the test. A dose of 370-400 MBq of Tc-99m Infecton given intravenously for an adult is recommended. Appropriate changes in dose for the children are required based on age or body weight. Anterior and posterior static whole body imaging is undertaken at approximately 1 and 4 hours and occasionally at 24 hours post injection, using a large field of view gamma camera peaked to 140 kev with a 15% window and a low energy all parallel hole collimator. Each spot image should have at least 500K count.

Biodistribution

On intravenous administration Tc-99m Infecton distributes throughout the body with a high uptake in the kidneys and moderate uptake in the liver and spleen. There is no bone marrow, muscle or bone uptake seen. The radiotracer remains in blood pool and with time reduction in this blood pool activity is seen. It is excreted by the kidneys to the urinary bladder. A site of bacterial infection shows a focal area of uptake. The delayed images with reduced blood pool activity make the lesions more obvious. In an abscess no uptake of

TC-99m Infecton is seen in the centre as it contains dead bacteria although the area surrounding the abscess where the living bacteria proliferate shows uptake [6,8].

Clinical Evaluation

Over 150 patients have been studied with Tc-99m Infecton at our centre. We have not observed any adverse effect from the intravenous injection of this radiotracer. Its role has been evaluated in skeletal, abdominal, endocardial, skin and soft tissue infections with encouraging results.

Although it is difficult always to confirm conclusively the presence or absence of living bacteria in the cases studied with Tc-99m Infecton, an attempt has been made to have a complete microbiological evaluation. In the cases where there was absence of adequate microbiological data, the clinical management and outcome analysis was taken as demonstrating bacterial infection, keeping in mind that the administration of antibiotic therapy could successfully eradicate the live bacteria.

The majority of work has been with skeletal infections involving the spine or lower limbs. The sensitivity, specificity and accuracy of 89%, 91% and 90% respectively was observed which is superior to Tc-99m HMPAO labelled leucocytes [8]. It is probably due to limited granulocyte turnover due to high pressure in infected vertebra or the relative physiological uptake of radiolabelled WBC in the bone marrow of neighbouring vertebral bodies as hypothesized [9]. The lack of bone marrow uptake unlike radiolabelled WBC imaging makes TC-99m Infecton an attractive approach. Besides there is always a need for a specific approach to detect bacterial infection in skeletal lesions as the antibiotic therapy is required over a long period of time.

An other group of patients evaluated are those with abdominal infection where a sensitivity, specificity and accuracy of 86%, 71% and 79% was seen [8]. Thus it can act as a valuable guide to distinguish the infected from non infected inflammatory bowel disease in turn facilitating appropriate therapy. Besides an abscess in relation to major organs of abdomen can be effectively discovered such as a psoas abscess (Fig 1). The role of Tc-99m

Infecton imaging to established. The lack of significant biliary excretion upto 4 hours makes it easy to detect active bacterial infection in the bowel. The results in cardiac and soft tissue infections have also been encouraging in small series reported [6,8].

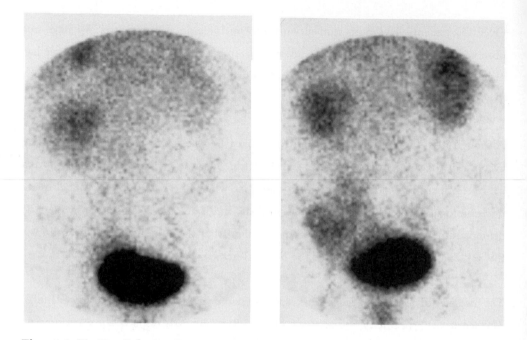

Figure 1. Tc-99m *Infection Image: Anterior view of abdomen at one hour p.i (left) and four hours p.i (right) in a case of Psoas abscess. There is increasing uptake in the lesion seen with time.*

It was observed that many cases with a negative Infecton scan had received antibiotic therapy before the study eradicating live bacteria in the targes site of this imaging. Using an appropriate categorisation for patients who had received antibiotic therapy prior to scan it is seen that an overall sensitivity, specificity and accuracy of 83%, 91% and 87% is obtained [8]. Thus for more meaningful Tc-99m Infecton scans, it is preferred to perform the test before starting or on the first day of antibiotic therapy and repeat if necessary later to see conversion from a positive to a negative image at the site of infection.

Dosimetry

The effective dose from the injection of Tc-99m Infecton was estimated to be about 4 mSv which is within WHO category II. The critical organ is urinary bladder.

Infection VS WBS Imaging

Although the imaging technique used for detecting infection in a department is dependent on many factors like local availability of facilities and expertise, it is seen that at present radiolabelled WBC scanning is the method of choice to image bacterial infection. An evaluation of Tc-99m Infecton in comparison with radiolabelled WBC has been done [6]. The concordance rate of the Tc-99m Infecton and radiolabelled leucocyte images was 68%. These images ranged over several clinical conditions, including skeletal, skin and soft tissue, abdominal and respiratory tract infection. In the study discordance between the white cell image and the Tc-99m Infecton image was noted in 32% of the total of 57 cases. Nine (50%) of these cases showing discordant results had positive Tc-99m Infecton scan but a negative WBC image and in the other nine (50%) with discordant results Tc-99m Infecton was negative whereas the WBC image was positive.

Eight out of nine cases of discordant results with Tc-99m Infecton being positive and Tc-99m WBC scan being negative were actually microbiologically true positive for infection. The classical situation of Tc-99m Infecton negative and WBC image positive is Crohn's disease where there is active inflammation but no bacterial infection. The other situations are sterile pouchitis and in situations mimicking osteomyelitis.

An interesting observation noted on the 18 patients reported with discordant results is that 11 of them were on antibiotics during imaging. Patients with a negative Tc-99m Infecton mage had been on therapy for significantly longer (19.6 days) than those with a positive Tc-99m Infecton image (8.8 days). Microbiological data suggests that this discrepancy is because antibiotic therapy has successfully eradicated live bacteria. Thus taking into accounts of the effects of antibiotic therapy, Tc-99m Infecton imaging gives higher sensitivity (84%), specificity (96%) and accuracy (90%) compared with white blood cell imaging (sensitivity 81%, specificity 77% and accuracy 79%) [6].

There are certain distinct advantages of Tc-99m Infecton over conventional methods of radiolabelled white cell imaging. Firstly Tc-99m Infecton does not require handling of blood or blood products during preparation, reducing the risk of needle injury, hepatitis B and HIV infection. Secondly, Tc-99m Infecton is packaged as a kit and is technically easier and less labour intensive than radioleballing white blood cells. Third, this method is independent of the white blood cell status of the patient and thus has a valuable advantage to identify bacterial infection in leucopeniic patients. Fourthly, it is a small molecule with potentially better tissue penetration than labelled white cells or antibodies. This may be important in areas such as an infected metal hip prothesis. Finally, because Tc-99m Infecton is not taken up by bone marrow, the agent can identify infection in the spine and proximal parts of the limbs.

Future Prospects

The use of radiolabelled quinolones in clinical practice is one example of the opening of the era of adding specificity to the usually sensitive nuclear medicine procedures in imaging infection and inflammation. However the clinical experience so far with this approach needs to be expanded with further comparison to other modalities like radiolabelled WBC scanning and radiological studies. A multicentric study is being initiated. Further use of Tc-99m Infecton will decide whether this will supplant, supplement or compliment the established methods of radiolabelled WBC imaging to detect bacterial infection.

It is seen that antibiotic therapy prior to imaging may lead to negative results. This needs further careful scrutiny as to whether effectiveness of antibiotic therapy can be decided on the changes on infection image from positive to negative in a patient with bacterial infection. It may also provide an opportunity to evaluate the presence of bacteria even before leucocyte migration to an infection site has taken place. The proof of principle that a radiolabelled antibiotic can target and image sites of bacterial infection may be extendable to the identification of fungal, protozoal and even viral infections in the future.

Summary

Most inflammation seeking radiopharmaceuticals target somewhere in the cascade of the inflammatory reaction, irrespective of the causative agent. Although the nuclear medicine techniques are sensitive, they often lacks specificity. To add specificity to the detection of bacterial infection Tc-99m labelled ciprofloxacin - Infecton was developed and evaluated. It showed its ability to detect bacterial infection in clinical situations with better sensitivity, specificity and accuracy than radiolabelled WBC. So far, no adverse effects are linked to Tc-99m Infecton imaging and the technique is easy. Successful antibiotic therapy prior to scan may lead to negative results. Thus Tc-99m Infecton imaging should be performed before antibiotic treatment or as soon as is practical after starting it and repeated if pyrexia persists.

Acknowledgements

We acknowledge the support of Commonwealth Scholarship Commission for Dr. Ravi Kashyap and the facilities provided by the St. Bartholomew's Foundation for research. The British Technology group have been of great help in patenting Tc-99m Infecton.

References

1] Solanki KK, Bomanji J, Siraj Q, et al. Tc-99m Infecton: a new class of radiopharmaceutical for imaging infection [abstract]. J Nucl Med 1993; 34:119P.
2] British National Formulary, March 1996; 31:257.
3] Tudor RG, Youngs DJY, Yoshioka K, et al. A comparison of the penetration of two quinolones into intra abdominal abscess. Arch Surg 1988; 123:1487-90.
4] Hooper DC, Wolfson JS, Ng EY, Schwartz MN. Mechanisms of action of and resistance to ciprofloxacin. Am J Med 1987; 82(supple 4A):12-20.
5] Riesbeck K, Siguardsson M, Leanderson T, Forsgren A. Superinduction of cytokine gene transcription by ciprofloxacin. J Immunol 1994; 153:343-52.
6] Vinjamuri S, Hall AV, Solanki KK, et al. Comparison of Tc-99m Infecton imaging with radiolabelled white cell imaging in the evaluation of bacterial infection. Lancet 1996; 347:233-5.
7] Jamu JK, Solanki KK, Britton KE. 99m Tc-Infecton: a new kit formulation [abstract]. Nucl Med Commun 1996; 17:285.
8] Vinjumari S, Hall A, Solanki K, et al. Use of 99m-Tc Infecton for localising bacterial infection imaging: clinical evaluation in 102 studies. Submitted for publication.
9] Becker W. The contribution of nuclear medicine to the patient with infection. Eur J Nucl Med 1995; 22:1195-211.

INDEX